Living with Vitality

Living with Vitality

The Role of the Life Force in Health & Disease

John Boulderstone

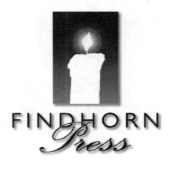

FINDHORN
Press

First published by Findhorn Press 2006

ISBN 10: 1–84409–071–X
ISBN 13: 978-1-84409-071-6

Edited by Kate Keogan
Cover design by Damian Keenan
Interior design by Pam Bochel

Printed by WS Bookwell, Finland

Published by
Findhorn Press
305a The Park, Findhorn
Forres IV36 3TE
Scotland, UK

tel 01309 690582/fax 690036
info@findhornpress.com
www.findhornpress.com

Contents

A poor man went to a wise man of a particular tribe and asked the following question:

'What are the parts within a body that go to support the person and, of these parts, which is the most important?'

The wise man replied:

'The parts are Physical Sensations, Thoughts, Feelings, Dreams and Ego.'

And each part boasted in turn, 'We support the person.'

But the Life Force said, 'Do not fool yourselves; I am the one that animates all of you and I alone am chief support to the person.'

But the parts would not believe the words of the Life Force. To demonstrate the truth, Life Force rose up and left the body, which then appeared to be dead, and returned five minutes later, re-animating the body, and said, 'There you are; that is proof that I am supreme.'

Thoughts said, 'What are you talking about? Nothing happened. I don't remember a thing.'

Feelings said, 'I felt something but I don't know what it was and it only lasted the shortest of time. Did you feel anything, Dreams?'

Dreams said, 'I think I fell asleep.' But Thoughts said, 'I thought you never slept,' and Dreams had to admit that this was probably the first time that he had.

Ego kept repeating that he was the best at everything and was no help to the discussion.

In the end, each part believed that they were the most important for there was no scientific proof to the contrary.

The poor man understood and became rich.

Adapted from the Prasna Upanishad

Foreword

Imagine you are walking past a casino, you look onto the ground and see a wad of twenty pound notes. No one is around, so you pick it up and count out the money: there is a thousand pounds. Enough for a holiday, perhaps.

Instead, you decide to go into the casino and put the money on a single number on the roulette wheel. The odds of winning are approximately 32 to 1 and that is what the casino pays out if your number comes up. Anyway, your number does come up and you now have an extra £32,000 pounds.

An hour ago, you were minding your own business and now you don't need to work for a year. This is a little too much to handle and so, in an attempt to get back to something normal, you put the whole amount on another 32 to 1 single number, really hoping to lose. However, your number comes up. Now your whole life has changed, you have just won over a million pounds. You feel weak, sick, stunned and confused all at the same time. Perhaps you could give the money away to your friends. You just want the feelings you are experiencing to stop – it wasn't even your thousand pounds in the first place – you should be happy, but it doesn't feel right.

Finally, in one last ditch effort to put everything right, you count out one thousand pounds and put the rest of the million pounds on the number zero. Reality is only one spin away. You can put the thousand pounds back where you found it and have a story to tell your grandchildren that no one will believe anyway. The wheel spins and, as the ball clanks around the wheel, you already know it will land in zero. You have won the casino and all the money in it. Now there is no escape.

This is the story of my life, but I didn't win money, I 'won' something more valuable. It started when I found I could heal twisted ankles and other strains. After this, I upped the stakes and found that phantom limb pain could be removed relatively easily. After this, I discovered the next level: the progression of the disease Multiple Sclerosis could be halted in its tracks. Finally, I realised that all illnesses are created by distortions in the flow of life force, and are therefore all susceptible to being cured by a healer able to work with this knowledge.

Every human being has the power to be a health millionaire and to live with vitality. This book is written to show you how.

Part 1: The True Nature of Health and Disease

Vitality is the key to health

You are responsible for your health – not your doctor, not your parents and not your children. When you accept that responsibility, you begin to have the power to change your health (and also that of others) for the better.

But what does it really mean to be healthy or ill? This book describes how to transform disease into health – or, to put it more accurately, how to use your vitality to get healthy and stay healthy regardless of how ill you may be at this moment in time.

Vitality is the key. Vitality is the spirit a boxer uses after he has been knocked down, as he gets up and goes on to win the fight. It is the spirit you have to use when you turn and face a chasing monster in a dream. And it is the spirit you use when confronted with any difficult or new situation. Your vitality informs you how to act in these difficult situations: do you tell the truth? Do you confront? Do you become the victim? Do you fight back? Having a strong vitality is essential to living healthily and overcoming disease.

Most people in the west believe that there is only one method of healing: that of western medicine. In reality, there are many other healing systems available to the sick person – such as acupuncture, spiritual healing, shiatsu and homeopathy, to name just a few. Each has its own, unique philosophy but all of these philosophies can be divided between just two categories: those which take account of your vitality (alternative therapies) and those which do not.

Vitality is a quality of living: having the energy to do what you want to do, to overcome your problems. Your vitality can be increased – or, to put it more accurately, the blocks that you put up and which depress your vitality can be removed. What happens if your vitality is increased? The answer is that *all* of your problems become smaller, whether they are health-related or not.

Vitality, like enthusiasm, can be contagious. When you see somebody is enthusiastic about something in their life, that enthusiasm can rub off on to you. This is how salesmen sell and how your friends get you to do things you might not truly want to do. You can get drawn into someone else's enthusiasm but it will always be just that: someone else's enthusiasm. If you do not fully share their world view, your sharing in their enthusiasm for something will be limited. If they view the world in an eccentric way, it will be more difficult for others to follow. Enthusiasm is one, generally positive form of vitality; vitality itself comes from within and can flow in many different directions.

Every therapy seeks to find a common language between patient and healer. This book explains that there is a common language, based on the flow of vitality. *You can alter the nature of your vitality because you can communicate with it.* In later chapters you will see how to change your vitality in order to overcome any disease.

Understanding how your vitality works is the key to understanding your health and therefore your happiness. You cannot separate one from the other. Some people say, 'Oh, I don't care about my health; I just want to be happy.' But not until you take on responsibility for your own health, and care about it, can you start to experience real happiness. For good health does not refer only to a functioning body: good health involves emotional, mental and spiritual wellbeing, too.

Warning: do not let the simplicity and obviousness of the observations presented in this book be a barrier to your understanding. People love complexity in their diseases – the more complex the better – for they believe this shows that they themselves are less likely to be part of the process. Yet health and healing become more attainable when responsibility for the illness is taken. Virtually all of my patients tell me how they believe they got their disease and how their doctors do not want to hear about this, but talk instead about bugs, germs, bad luck and how disease is a complicated process. Their doctors may tell them that no cure is possible at the moment, but that there may be one within fifty years. From the viewpoint of western medicine this may be true. There are other ways of looking than through the eyes of western medicine.

The science of vitality

Virtually every single disease will succumb to an increase in vitality. The only ones that will not are those in which the very blueprint of the person is distorted.

Vitality *is life-enthusiasm.*

Vital force *is vitality flowing through the body. Vital force is also called* **life force**.

Most of the world's health-systems make use of the vital force. However, the health system with which most of us in the west have grown up – that of western medicine – does not. Even so, life expectancy in the west has increased and is still increasing, and many diseases have been eradicated. Does this mean that vitality and vital force are not necessary to healing? Or that taking them into account is not so important? Take a look at the next section to find out.

Measurement

After the Renaissance, science began to see the body as a mechanical object. The vital force, spirit and soul were seen as the domain of religion, and problems involving them were dealt with by the clergy. Disease was increasingly believed to be caused by external influences and not the product of God's judgement. This may not have been true of the ordinary person, however, who still saw an illness as the just desserts of a bad act. Indeed, even today, some people will say they know that the reason they are ill is that they have done something to cause their illness. As one of my patients recently said: 'I was an emotional mess, I knew I was behaving badly... something had to give and it did. I got MS.'

On the whole, doctors became scientists while the clergy looked after the soul. As time has gone by, this division has become more and more distinct. Of course, there are occasional crossovers because any artificial division of nature will always fail to be one hundred percent complete. Psychologists often stray into work with the soul, and some exorcisms in the church may well be better served by psychotherapists.

Another problem with science, and therefore with western medicine, is that it does not seem to recognize anything which cannot be measured. Not only must everything be measured, but it must be measured *objectively*. The gold standard of testing in medicine, the double-blind trial, goes to extremes in this quest for objectivity. In so doing, many human qualities that cannot be measured are ignored, some of them deliberately. For example, love is a powerful stimulant in many ways. It has been shown to speed up the recovery of people with various illnesses. But love is not measurable and so western medicine usually dismisses it – at least, it is not generally mentioned in textbooks on nursing the sick – yet I am sure that most people are aware of its importance.

Measuring the immeasurable

One of the strange anomalies within western medicine is the fact that it finds it hard even to measure health. This gives rise to ridiculous situations where a surgeon may say, 'The operation was a complete success but the patient died of pneumonia a week later.' The chances are that the patient succumbed to the pneumonia because their vitality had been depressed by the operation. If their vitality could have been monitored before and after the operation, a different outcome could have been achieved.

Where the human body is concerned, western medicine actually has a very hard time in defining terms which at first glance appear easy to understand. This is because western medicine does not really know what life is. Just look at the problems it has in defining the absence of life: death. Does death occur when the heart stops or when brain activity ceases? When does death occur? This question is crucial to understanding life, yet doctors must often refer to the law-court when there is disagreement between themselves and their patient's family.

The ability to measure something can be useful. But to deny the usefulness of vitality or love because you cannot measure them will cause everyone's health to suffer. Life expectancy may have increased due to the efforts of western medicine, but that does not mean that the health of most people has improved as well. Without bringing vitality into the equation, you will never be able to tell if 'average health' has increased or not. Certainly, more people are alive today than would be if western medicine did not exist, but it can also be argued that general health is poorer. Many more children, nowadays, are unable to deal with dust, cope with dairy products or easily throw off common childhood illnesses. Is this progress? If not, whose responsibility is it?

There appears to be more auto-immune disease around today than ever before because we are neglecting the most important part of our health: our vital force. The strength of each individual depends on their vitality, yet we ignore this and isolate the body. There are cardiac specialists, pulmonary specialists, kidney specialists etc. – these doctors all specialize in parts. Yet we are not just a collection of parts. Any one part of us that is not functioning correctly is but a symptom and a reflection of a disordered vitality or vital force. How is it that this western, scientific model of reality has insinuated itself so completely into the western psyche that we cannot envisage any other way of being?

Although vital force, like love, cannot be measured objectively, many people feel it in themselves and in others. And even though it cannot be measured in particular units of size or time, it can still be measured with certainty and clarity, for there are other ways of measuring besides that of the scientific model – we can 'get the measure' of it. If two people were to present themselves to you, I suspect that even without training you would be able to tell if their vitality was similar or different. If you think about the people you know, there will be some whose vitality stands out as being greater than that of others. This is just a simple test but one which has huge consequences if used in the right way.

So, although science can only prove things according to its own, objective model, this is not the only way. There are some things known to us as individuals that do not need to be backed up by science -indeed, science probably *cannot* back them up. We may base our whole life on concepts that, according to science, are 'impossible'. Homeopathy is a case in point. After I took a prescribed homeopathic pill, I had a reaction that gave me a huge boost of energy (vitality) which was sustained over several days. During this time, the frequently recurring headaches I had gone to see the homeopath about disappeared, and I felt much better *in myself.* All that western medicine had been able to offer me were painkillers. The active ingredient in the single homeopathic pill I took was not of a scientifically measurable quantity. Science says that there was no active ingredient, but the effect was something I will never forget. It was on the basis of this one pill that I changed my life. I knew then that science did not have all the answers. We all know a lot more than can be proven by science.

Angela's cat

Angela had a cat who was exclusive – by this I mean a cat who was only interested in one person. When Angela was ill, she would come and sit on her bed every day, without exception, making herself comfortable and just being present. The day Angela died, the cat came into the room, looked at the body and, for the first time ever, went and sat on Angela's husband's bed. I am sure there are many possible reasons for this but life force must figure somewhere in the explanation.

Suppression

Why do we entrust something as important as our health (and therefore our happiness) to science? This is the question that goes to the heart of the human condition. Western medicine works – or it appears to work. However, most of western medicine is concerned with suppression. For example, if a patient presents with eczema, the first medicine that is tried is a steroid cream. This ignores the cause of the eczema but, more often than not, the damaged skin gets better. When someone has a headache, painkillers are generally prescribed – again ignoring the reason the headache developed in the first place. The painkillers modify the pain, sometimes even taking it away completely; a connection is made between the pill or cream prescribed by the doctor and the alleviation of symptoms. This is something with which you cannot argue. Who wants to suffer? Science can prove that western medicine works but only insofar as it treats symptoms; it ignores the complete health, or vitality, of the patient.

Here is a genuine case: a patient had bad eczema on her legs and went to her GP. He prescribed two different creams, one to use at night and one during the day, for up to a month. She duly followed his advice and, while the eczema began to clear, she started to get ill with nausea and exhaustion (basically, reduced vitality). After various tests, Mrs X was referred to hospital with liver disease, diagnosed as a 'side effect' of the eczema creams.

What happens to the health of the patient after it has been suppressed by western medicine? On first sight, because the presenting complaint improves, it appears to the doctor that they have a successful outcome – until, that is, you bring vitality into the equation. The case described above is reasonably dramatic; what if, instead of liver disease, she had developed something less dramatic – headaches, for example? The emergence of the headaches might never be associated with the eczema creams. They may disappear after the creams have been discontinued but there is no guarantee that this will happen. I have seen many cases where new symptoms have appeared after western medicine has been given and these new symptoms have not gone away, even when the medicine was stopped. An energy-based therapy is usually the only way to put a stop to this spiralling bad health.

We will talk about this later. For now, it is important to see that the symptom which the body was producing, namely the eczema, has been taken away and prevented from occurring. This is true for all suppression: the main symptom is actually overpowered by the drug and not allowed free expression. The consequences of this on a person's complete health are always detrimental.

Cause or response?

The way in which people describe the cause of their symptoms is rarely accurate. People's view of what happens to them is limited, and this in itself is a problem. They usually talk about the cause of their illness as being an event outside themselves. For instance, they may say that a headache was caused by flashing lights, a loud noise, or eating chocolate; in reality, the true cause is their *response* to that event. This can be shown to be true in that not everyone will develop a headache when exposed to exactly the same situation or event. The cause of all disease is never an event: rather, it is an inappropriate *response* to an event. (If an event were the true cause, you would only have to avoid it and the symptoms would go away.) This inappropriate response is individual to the patient. It is dependent upon the history of the individual and is governed by his or her vitality.

All disease has a cause if you take the life force into account. If you have no concept of the life force, illness and disease can seem to appear 'from out of the blue'. What else in life happens without a cause? Nothing. So why is disease any different? The answer, of course, is that it is not different; there is always a cause for disease but it is not always obvious.

The vital force has a memory and responds in a similar way each time it receives the same stimulus. This is to say that our vitality creates vital paths. Attached to a vital path can be everything that we ever experience. Thoughts, emotions and physical sensations are all part of the vital force package. This explains how memories can be stimulated with the flow of vitality.

We all have locked inside us responses to events which can have strong physiological expressions. Just imagine sinking your teeth into the sourest lemon you have ever tasted. If you do that now, it does not take long for saliva to build up in your mouth even though you are only using your imagination. But what would it be like if, locked inside your head, you had an event that was horrendous? Every time you connected with that event, your body would relive your initial response to it.

A common problem that people come to see me with is panic attacks. They have usually been to their doctor first, who will have prescribed an anti-depressant or some other drug. The drug may work for a while, but the attacks soon start up again and the patient ends up coming to see someone like me. The problem is that the person has experienced a stressful event and then not completely dealt with it; the panic attack is his/her way of trying to relive the event in an unconscious attempt to process it fully. Whenever something happens which in some way mimics the original trauma, the body tries to relive the initial event. The drugs just distract the person or alter their mental state to confuse them; this actually slows down the process of cure. While the 'problem' may appear to be whatever it is that triggers the panic attack, the *real* problem is the suppressed trauma. Once this is known, cure is possible – otherwise the patient will be forever chasing the triggers. The prescription of drugs will make cure more difficult to achieve. What needs to be addressed is why the vitality disappeared when it was most needed.

Vitality can slip away easily when responsibility is relinquished. On the physical level, the taking of a single painkiller or anti-depressant does not, usually, greatly affect the vitality, and it is more than likely that the vitality will recover fully in time. However, on the mental level, even taking a single painkiller means that the patient has bought into the idea that pain is to be avoided, rather than seeing the pain as a message of distress to be listened to. Once listened to, the vital force has the power to heal all disease.

Vital force throughout the world

The majority of people throughout the world believe in, and use the existence of, the vital force as a powerful ally in staying alive and healthy, but it is often given another name. Christianity calls it the Holy Spirit. There is no debate within Christianity as to the existence or otherwise of the Holy Spirit because scientific proof is not required. In Judaism, vital force is called *Ruach*, the breath of God. In China, it is called *chi* and is the basis of acupuncture, Tai Chi and art. In India, it is called *prana* and is the basis of Ayurvedic medicine and yoga. In Japan, it is important in the martial arts – judo, kendo, aikido and karate – where it is referred to as *ki*. It is worth bearing in mind that warriors practising the martial arts, and who put their lives at risk, would be unlikely to bother with the vital force unless it made a real difference to their skills.

The existence of the vital force is taken for granted in most cultures. Only in the West is there a question mark around it, and even then only within a portion of the scientific community (the reason being that it cannot yet be measured). However, you do not need to wait until its existence can be proved before you use it to regain full health for yourself and others.

Vitality theory

> *I use the word 'healing' to mean sorting out the vitality of a sick person so that they can overcome their disease. Alternative therapies can be defined as those which use the vital force in this way.*

Vital force – divided

Everything we do or think or feel has vitality associated with it. That vitality moves in a certain way, sometimes strongly, at other times less so. When it is strong, we have reserves which allow us to look at the world and see our options. Generally, the more options we have, the healthier we are. However, when we are in conflict with ourselves, our vital force will be pulled in at least two different directions at the same time. In this case, the vital force will be divided and will not flow as efficiently as it could. In this way, illness creeps in to show us the way to health.

Imagine that you have just won the lottery: your mind will be excited by all the new possibilities that have opened up, and you will have very little vitality left to do the mundane things in life like eating and sleeping. When the vital force has become divided, and this division is left unresolved for long enough, a physical illness will always result. In fact, disease can be defined as *a division of the vital force*. From this follows a definition of health: *the smooth, uninterrupted flow of vitality or vital force*.

Vital force – reduced

Vital force flows through us and we have the power to alter its flow. We can slow it down. We usually do this because we need to learn something. The next time our vital force flows down this particular vital path, we will have more control over our senses and feelings. When our vital force slows down, we will notice that our breathing also slows down and that our options become fewer. This can often be seen when somebody is learning something new. As an example of this, you often hear yoga teachers telling their class to keep breathing because, as they go a little further into a posture, it becomes important to be aware of what is happening physically (and energetically). The life force is slowed down and the breathing goes the same way. In yoga, there is an exercise called *pranayama* which is most often translated as 'breathing exercise'; it is more correctly translated as 'energy exercise'. This shows how closely connected energy is to the breath.

You can also consciously change how your vitality flows because you can communicate with it. It talks to you in a similar language to that of your dreams. If you have the power to create the necessary images, you can modify many physiological effects. Most people are aware that through using internal imagery you can modify your blood pressure, lower your anxiety levels and even change your temperature within seconds. The only thing that holds you back from using your vitality to its fullest extent and being completely healthy is the correct understanding and knowledge of how it operates.

Vitality is in every act you make. I have occasionally seen people who have virtually no life force and yet they are walking around and (from a distance, at least) appear quite normal. Up close, though, you can see that they have no resistance: they will not argue with you; they do not do or create anything. Very often they have pain but they do not respond to it; they tend to take to their bed. These people can live a long time but, in essence, they are the walking dead. Their vitality has been taken up by unresolved problems from the past.

Part 2: How to Get Ill

All disease has a single cause and that cause is inner conflict.

Vitality, or life force, flows through everyone. Even if it is impossible to understand the life force fully, we ignore it at our peril. If it were to flow through us without being diverted or restricted, we would be perfect. The resistances which we put up to it make us human. The stronger the resistance, the stronger we feel – except that, because of this apparent strength, we also get ill and we forget what is really important.

There is no fixed structure through which the life force flows; the life force comes first and lies beneath all structure. This is what makes it unique and exceedingly difficult to describe. Any structure you can envisage may be superimposed on it; the meridians of the acupuncturist, chakras of the Ayurvedic physician and even the three worlds of the shaman are all valid. None of these is wrong but neither do they contain the whole story. The life force transcends every description and definition. This is why the life force can never get completely blocked and never stops. It also means that all therapies have the potential to work, even if their philosophies contradict each other. When therapies really work, they always work in the same way: by resolving the person's inner conflict – the cause of all disease. As soon as the inner conflict which caused the disease is resolved, health will follow.

Inner conflict can sometimes be expressed in words but this is not always the case. It actually exists as an energetic conflict; it is this that all therapies try to resolve, whether or not they are aware of the fact.

When there is inner conflict in our lives, the vitality becomes divided between the conflicting parts of our being. When vitality gets divided, physical symptoms will result unless the conflict is removed. This is because the physical body is a reflection of the flow of vitality and is governed by it. Nor is it just the physical body that draws on the flow of vital force – our thoughts and emotions, all of our senses, and even our personality are under its influence.

The best therapy will be one which directly accesses the restrictions and diversions created in the life force by the individual. The Boulderstone Technique of Life Force Healing is one such therapy.

Susceptibility

The majority of people believe that viruses and bacteria are the cause of illness and disease. This is only true insofar as one disregards the vitality of the patient. I am well aware that viruses and bacteria exist and appear to cause problems, but are they actually the *cause* of disease? The answer is not as clear-cut as one might think. Certainly, from a life force perspective, diseases are only caused by distorted life force, while viruses and bacteria put in an appearance after the event.

I am not alone in this view. Antoine Bechamp claimed that Louis Pasteur, the founder of germ theory, stole his ideas, oversimplified them and thereby created problems. His followers claim that this oversimplification has shaped modern medicine to the detriment of everyone's health. In the end, even Pasteur acknowledged Bechamp.

Pasteur believed that disease comes from bugs, external to the body, which have to be fought off because they can get anyone. Bechamp, on the other hand, believed that the harmful micro-organisms found in diseased people mutated *within the person* as a result of an unhealthy environment. Bechamp's ideas have not been disproved. Indeed, they fit well with the theories of all life force therapies. In contrast, Pasteur's ideas only make sense if the life force is ignored.

Pasteur's ideas have given rise to the pharmaceutical industry – just as they should, if they were correct. However, if the ideas were built on false premises, the consequence would be that real health issues would never be properly addressed. New drugs would continually be needed as unhealthy people, denied the expression of easy diseases (e.g. through mild, childhood diseases which have been suppressed by vaccination), create ever more complex micro-organisms to co-habit in the world. This contrast between Pasteur and Bechamp is perfectly reflected today in the different perspectives of western medicine and alternative medicine.

Therapists that work with the life force believe that you can only get ill if your vitality isn't functioning properly. It is then that the appropriate bugs come along to exploit the weakness.

If a particular bacteria or virus were solely responsible for a particular disease, everyone exposed to it would succumb to that disease. This does not happen. Some people have the ability to resist the disease, even though they have been exposed to its bugs. The ability to resist or avoid a disease is the role of the vitality or life force. Of course, the immune system plays its part but the immune system is just the physical aspect of the life force. The immune system can actually be transformed in an instant. It can be strengthened in seconds through therapies like the Boulderstone Technique, homeopathy and kinesiology. It can be weakened in seconds by shock – both emotional (e.g. receiving bad news) or physical (e.g. an accident). Most people think of health as a slowly improving or slowly worsening state of the body. This is materialistic thinking. Once you are into the realms of energy, you realize that changes can happen very quickly, even if the physiological changes in the body occur more slowly than the changes in its life force.

The role of every disease is to bring your attention to the absence of vitality, to show you the way back to health.

Other so-called causes of disease – such as pollution, accidents, bad luck, acts of God, inherited bad genes and random attacks – can also be explained in terms of vitality. A weakened life force makes you not only more susceptible to these 'causes' in the first place but also to suffering bad effects from them.

An accident can only happen if your awareness is withdrawn and you do not see the event coming. Vitality has the power to prevent accidents because the more vital you are, the more your focus is outward and ready to respond and adapt to any new situation. The more symptoms you have, the more you focus on them and the more your attention is taken up. Your vitality is also essential to recovering when problematic things happen.

Vitality as a measure of health

The vitality of an individual can be seen as a measure of health for that person. The same can be said for any living entity. Indeed, anything which can be considered to have a life-cycle will have vitality and therefore its health can be measured. (For example, an ant colony, any community, a tree, an orchard, a government, a country or even the entire earth.)

Pollution may be a big problem but essentially it comes from not understanding the vitality of the environment. Stopping a major polluter without looking at the vitality of the environment is much the same as removing or suppressing a symptom in a person and not looking at its cause. The base problem still exists but, by the time it shows itself again, the problem will be worse.

Inherited 'bad' genes, giving rise to various congenital conditions, may be the one thing we cannot do much about, except to learn how to work with what we have been given. Increasing our vitality always leads to a better quality of life, whatever our starting point. Gene therapy will not be a solution unless it takes the life force into account, for the life force will just re-create the underlying problem until it is addressed. The same is true for stem cell therapy. Conversely, if the life force distortion is sorted out, stem cell therapy will work.

Illness can only come about because our vitality gets reduced. This is discussed in the next section.

Discrete living-realms

To understand how we create a reduced or divided vital force, we need to look at the way in which we view the world and ourselves.

Most adults think of themselves as individuals, separate from others, yet this viewpoint lies at the heart of the problem. What is needed is an understanding of what a person really is. In the physical body there are many micro-organisms living and going about their daily business. Without them we could not survive: their activities are essential to human life; they break down food and so allow us to gain essential nutrients. But the relationship works both ways; without our bodies these micro-organisms would not live. They are so connected to our existence that in one sense they are a real part of us. Physically, then, we are not as individual as we may think.

It is similar for the mind. We may think that we are just one person but, in reality, we are made up of a lot of different egos (our personality is the sum of all of our egos). This does not mean that we are schizophrenic or suffering from multiple personality disorder but, again, we are not as individual as we may think.

If we look at every 'living' thing from the ant to the Earth, we will see that it does not exist in isolation.

In life we all have to take on many roles: spouse, parent, child, sibling, co-worker, boss, neighbour, stranger, for example. All of these roles carry with them different sets of values and rules to live by. Some of them may be conflicting. We might not even be conscious of the different values or how we swap in and out of different roles. It is perfectly possible for them to coexist and for us not to be aware of them. Only when they come into conflict with each other would we notice them. For example, you might be very liberal in your ideas concerning censorship and maintain that all censorship is a bad thing but, when your six-year-old daughter is confronted with some pornographic images, you notice that the liberal and parent egos are in conflict. Or it may be the case that at work your boss might tell a racist joke and you might laugh, whereas in any other situation you would not.

When you think of yourself as an individual, you have moved into a discrete living-realm – the land of the ego. This isolated place is responsible for the fantastic success we have had as a species but is also the birthplace of all our illness. Being isolated within a realm keeps us from viewing the whole and thereby creates inner conflict. Without these realms we would revert to being animals: with them we create our illnesses, dissatisfactions and emotional upsets.

Although these realms are created by each of us, individually, we are aided in the process by our families, our education and the people around us. Even though the life force flows through them, every realm has, at its core, a conflict. When we become aware of the conflict, we are forced to resolve it or become ill. Sometimes, we even prefer to become ill. Even the social lies about being well when we are not come about because of a conflict between different realms.

Realms of every kind are infectious; you only have to say to someone, 'Isn't it a lovely day?' and they could be sucked into a new realm.

The beginning of a realm is the word. You cannot comprehend the universe in its entirety yet you give it a name. This limiting, by the word, is the beginning of all illness. But life force still flows through everything even if it has a name. Life force is not comprehended by anything limited. I can feel this life force and teach anyone who has the desire to feel it also. This is because life force flows through everyone. When you become aware of the life force within yourself then you realize you are not just a body and a mind; you realize your true nature and then all illness is healed. Gospel according to St John (my own interpretation)

Even a word is a realm. It is designed to convey a meaning. But we can only guess that the meaning which we want to convey by that word is actually understood in the way we intend it. So, when we use a word, the person receiving it will probably understand it in a slightly differently way from how it was meant. Conflict will eventually follow.

Also, as each realm is limited, it will fail to describe the whole of the universe completely, for the universe will always be bigger than any realm we can imagine.

Our egos come to believe that the limited structures which they have created constitute everything. And here are more grounds for inner conflict. This is the current situation with orthodox medicine, where some of its practitioners believe that there simply is no other form of medicine.

The life force still flows through realms, but it existed before any realm was created.

Each ego lives in its own, discrete living-realm and is waiting to take its turn on stage. Each one believes that it is on its own, is unique and the real you. Sometimes you can see this when you find yourself reacting differently to the same person in the same situation, depending on which 'hat' you are wearing – or which ego is being displayed.

When you move into a discrete living-realm, it becomes your whole world. Everything you see will reflect that realm or be coloured by the perspective of that particular ego. For example, when you are pregnant you may notice all the other pregnant women, the articles in magazines about pregnancy and everything that relates to babies, although before that you barely noticed them. If you get stuck in a particular realm, it may lead to obsession. On television some years ago, someone was featured who loved Christmas so much that they created a room in the house where it was always Christmas, with decorations and a tree surrounded by presents all year round. This person was stuck in one discrete living-realm.

Many patients have come along for a consultation with me in a kind of depression where all they can see in the world around them is chaos, death and destruction. They do not know how to carry on living in such an evil world. After one treatment session, they feel so much better that they start to see the world quite differently.

Suddenly they notice how beautiful the world is around them. They realize how much they love their family and friends, how much hope and potential there is. What has changed? They have been released from the prison of their own making so that they can expand beyond the limitations of the one living-realm in which they were previously stuck.

The landscape of a dream is a discrete living-realm. When you are inside it, very often, you believe it is your whole world and, as such, it will be a reflection of your health.

The realms as the basis for inner conflict

We change from one realm to another all the time, each of them being governed by a different ego. In themselves they are an attempt to make our lives easier. Because we cannot remain comfortably in any one realm indefinitely, we will have conflicting values (if two realms share the same values then they are actually the same realm).

The ability to move from one realm to another is the real test of health. We need our separate egos – we cannot just get rid of them – but the more easily we can move from one to another, the healthier we are. Sometimes there is an easy transition between realms: sometimes it is more difficult. For example, the transition between work and 'home and the kids' can be difficult for some people. Bars fill up at the end of a working day with the people in them making a transition from one realm to another.

You create your realms as you need to and will stay healthy as long as you can move from one to another smoothly and easily. The difficulty lies in facing contradictory values between the realms that you have created. This is the only cause of stress. When two opposing values co-exist, we will experience inner conflict. It is this inner conflict that will go on to cause illness and disease if it remains unresolved.

As people grow older they tend to prefer to stay in the realms they know and are less prepared to shift their values and move from one realm to another. This results in the grumpiness associated with older people. Shock comes about when we cannot move quickly enough from one realm to another and so we take values from one realm into another in which they are inappropriate. When people tend to stick in the realms they are used to and become more entrenched, they are more easily shocked.

Carrying inner conflict is a recipe for problems. Everything that is experienced will have the potential for dispute and leads to a breeding ground for bacteria and viruses. These organisms can help by causing a disturbance in the conflicting realms, thus breaking up the status quo and allowing transformation. Traditionally, getting ill would ensure a spell in bed – this allowed people to let go of all the roles of the personality, to just 'be themselves' for a while, allowing them to sort out the internal conflicts before emerging recovered. However, these short, sharp, acute illnesses are increasingly being suppressed and avoided (e.g. by antibiotics or by vaccination), with the result that the need for the curative presence of illness can build up. Eventually, a far more serious, chronic diseased state becomes likely.

The energy behind the disease

It is important to clarify at this point that disease is not a state of mind but the result of vitality that has been divided or reduced. But, whilst there is a direct connection between disordered thinking and a disease, it is possible to change the thought and still leave the disease in place. It is the vital energy behind the disordered thinking that has to change in order to cure the disease. This is where the Boulderstone Technique is so effective (see *Part 5: The Boulderstone Technique of Life Force Healing*).

Similar energetic blocks in different people do not necessarily result in the same illness. Many different factors influence which illness will be suffered. The life force is affected by both individual and cultural factors on its way to the nameable disease. For example, breast cancer has a relatively higher incidence in the West compared to stomach cancer which is more common in the East. One example of different susceptibilities in different people concerns how emotions may be felt in different parts of the body by different individuals and different nationalities. When asked to point to the part of their body where emotions come from, different people from around the world have been known to point to their head, heart, liver, solar plexus or guts. Unresolved emotional issues, for these people, will affect their physical health in the areas pointed to. It is important to remember that the emotional and mental states do not have a direct effect on the physical body, as many people believe: both the emotion and the physical body are affected by the vitality.

The deeper the inner conflict and the more distorted the life force, the harder it will be to remove and the greater the resulting disease. There is also a hierarchy of symptoms. Colds, with relatively minor and transient symptoms, are easy to catch because the inner conflict behind the susceptibility is general in nature and thus also easier to catch. More serious diseases are usually more difficult to catch as the type of conflict involved is more specific to the individual. For example, if you believe your country is about to be invaded, the resulting affect on your life force could cause you to have a major illness, which may take a long time to develop. If the threat didn't materialize and diminished in your eyes, the illness would not come into existence for you. On the other hand, if you had issues around boundaries, the illness would develop a lot more quickly.

Most people know that it is actually possible to put off being ill if it is absolutely necessary. Schoolteachers often do this towards the end of the academic year. Somehow, if you use enough force, you can create a barrier to succumbing to an illness. It may be temporary, it may not, but it can be done. How is this done? If illness were solely the result of bugs then this phenomenon would not be possible. Of course, the answer is dependent on our vitality and how we use it. When we have learnt to use our vitality fully, we can head off illness. When we cannot use it at all, we can instantly succumb to any illness.

If an illness is put off and not discharged, the pressure of it gets greater until it overwhelms the barrier. Then the illness will come on at a much greater speed.

How vitality gets reduced; the consequences

Inner conflict causes loss of vitality.

It is easy to reduce your vitality and so become more susceptible to illness. Telling a simple lie, for example, will divide your vital force. This happens because you are holding on to the truth and, at the same time, have to keep track of the lie. A fork in the flow of your vital force has been created; this fork results in conflict each time you become aware of the possibilities. The consequences are definite physiological changes which can be picked up by a lie detector. Whenever we create inner conflict, our vitality always gets reduced.

Along with the Bible, one of the most important books on how to live without inner conflict, and therefore with full vitality, comes out of India and was written over 1,500 years ago by Patanjali. This book is not a series of rules, like the Ten Commandments; it is more about the causes of inner conflict and the way to resolve them. Patanjali states that there are only five causes of inner conflict: *prejudice, attachment, aversion, I-am-ness,* and *fear of endings.* Patanjali believes that, if you can see these five causes for what they are, you will not get ill. Let's take a brief look at each in turn and try to understand how they can reduce our vitality and hence lead to illness.

Patanjali says that **prejudice** is the first cause of inner conflict and is also the basis of the other four. The word 'prejudice' comes from the Latin *praeiudicium* (*prae* meaning 'before' and *iudicium* meaning 'sentence', from *iudex,* 'a judge'). Therefore prejudice refers to passing judgement before all the facts are in. If you do this, you are liable to make a mistake which will lead to loss of vitality. For example, say you cross the road without looking, having already assumed the road to be clear. Sooner or later you are going to experience a catastrophic loss of vitality!

But this is a little one-dimensional. Judgements are made on the basis of many factors. For example, even the apparently simple decision over which coat to wear when going out requires you to decide what the weather is like. If the weather changes, will you have to carry the coat? Will the colours and style conflict? Is it appropriate in the social setting? What is the state of the coat? But all these decisions are made without really thinking them through. Eventually you come up with a 'yes' or 'no' – the judgement. Now, as long as you remained open to all possibilities then there was no prejudice. But, if you decided right at the beginning that you were going to take the coat anyway, there is a lot of scope for problems to arise and vitality to be lost – especially if you are at a black-tie do and you are carrying around your old duffle coat which you were going to put on the guy next November. Prejudice carries with it much unforeseen potential for loss of vitality to occur.

Attachment, the second of Patanjali's causes of inner conflict, is the inability to let go. Marx said that 'all property is theft' and this is essentially what Patanjali is saying. This same concept exists in Christianity, when it is said that 'it is easier for a camel to pass through the eye of a needle than it is for a rich man to enter heaven'. (Heaven being, for our purposes, the equivalent of perfect health.) The Buddha also said that the basis of suffering is attachment. Holding on to something which you believe you own reduces your vitality. The truth is that you come into the world with nothing and you leave with nothing. The reality of holding on to something occurs internally. When something you feel you own gets lost, destroyed or stolen, it can feel devastating, depending on how close your attachment to it was. But if, internally, you see the true value of your possessions then no vitality will be lost in trying to keep hold of them. No one is saying that you have to give away everything you own, just that there are consequences in believing that you 'own' anything in the first place.

Aversion is very similar to attachment except that it works in the opposite direction. While attachment is about holding on to something, aversion is about pushing something away. In our culture, pain is considered to be something to be avoided at all costs – whether it is physical, emotional or mental pain. Let's take an everyday example: whenever you leave a particular task to the last moment, some sort of aversion is going on. As soon as the task is completed, however, you feel relief, indicating that the original 'pain' was showing you the way forward. Continuing to avoid pain leads to serious problems.

Painkillers stop or slow down the healing process. Aversion to remembered pain will always maintain distress. Post-traumatic Stress Disorder is a good example of this, where reliving the original cause, *with awareness*, completely removes the problem.

The next cause of inner conflict, according to Patanjali, is **I-am-ness** or **egotism.** This is the belief that you are supreme. It is a state which is much more common than one might imagine. From small children having a tantrum to the boss of a company throwing his or her weight around, we very often believe that we can do whatever we want. This is fine when we are completely aware of everyone around us who is going to be affected but, as soon as we remove our awareness, problems and inner conflict will arise.

Actually, our power is always limited to the world as we see it but we think that that world is the whole universe.

Patanjali's fifth and final cause of inner conflict and loss of vitality is **fear of endings**. In all probability, the one fear which everyone has at some time in their life is a fear of death. Having a fear of death actually means that we are not aware of what our own life truly is. Death can be a great source of lack of vitality! And not just for the dead but also for the living. People who believe that they are just a body (and there are many) fear death the most since, to them, death means annihilation. If you know yourself as the SELF, the part of you that is beyond personality, then you will never have a problem with endings, or any fear of death, and there will be no inner conflict. (See *Understanding Death.*)

Breaks in consciousness (BIC)

Coupled with inner conflict and the resulting split in the vitality is a situation which I call a break-in-consciousness or BIC. When the vitality splits – as in the case of telling a lie, for example – at least one path will have a dead end. This means that, as the awareness travels down this path and encounters the dead end, there will be a point when the awareness doesn't know where to go. This is a break in consciousness. It is a natural occurrence when learning something new but also comes about when you reach a point you feel you can't or don't want to go beyond.

Moreover, when you are pulled in two different directions through inner conflict, it is difficult to keep track of all the possibilities. Eventually you have to give up on one path; this path that you have given up will end in a break in consciousness. When you relive this path, through following a similar activity at some point in the future, you will encounter the BIC.

Although everyone experiences BICs, they most often occur when there is a change in level – either metaphorically or actually, since the mind sees everything as a metaphor. (For example, you go upstairs to retrieve something but halfway up the stairs you realize that you have forgotten what it was that you wanted.) A BIC will only occur when there is unresolved inner conflict (which includes learning experiences); even so, you might not be aware of the original conflict – it may well be forgotten in the past. This is because the energetic pathways which form are more significant than the event which took place. 'Irrational' fear is a good example of what happens when there is energetic learning but the original event which established the fear has been forgotten. You encounter a BIC whenever you forget something. A person suffering from an Obsessive-Compulsive disorder would come across BICs all the time.

A break in consciousness is not a punishment but rather the inevitable consequence of not resolving an inner issue. The more distracted you are, the more inner conflicts you have and the less healthy you are.

Levels / metaphors

Understanding how dreams work is a key to understanding the science of vitality. For example, when I need to go to the toilet in the middle of the night, I will often dream of a fire. This is my dream code. Somehow dreaming of a fire is meant to make me think of ways of putting the fire out and urinating on it is wired into my consciousness. This method of using symbols is common to both dreams and to vitality and is also picked up in our language.

If you are 'heartbroken', you may well have experienced grief of some sort but it may actually affect your physical heart. Likewise, being 'sick to your stomach' over an emotional issue sometimes causes vomiting or other digestive problems. In all probability, everyone has experienced this sort of thing at some time in their life and yet it is ignored by medical science because it is difficult to measure.

The vital force moves in its vital channels; these channels are not arbitrary nor are they fixed like the blood vessels. Instead, they follow whatever constructs have been created by the individual. So, if you ignore the remembered pain experienced in your heart because of a love affair that went wrong, you may well create two vital channels – one ending in a BIC in your physical heart and another that bypasses your heart. How many years need to pass before a surgeon gives you a heart bypass operation is dependent on how often the channels are used. There will always be a correlation between your illness and your internal representation of yourself as defined by your vital channels. You may encounter a specific bacterium or virus but these are always secondary to the loss of vitality caused by inner conflict.

How we learn

Stick or carrot.

The vital channels which create the internal representation we have of ourselves are unique to us. Having said that, because there are fundamental similarities between the people within a particular culture or social group, the channels created within each individual resemble those of others within the group. This is why we relate more easily to people who have had similar experiences to our own. It is not the experience that is important but the vital channels that are created as a result of it.

The vital channels which are laid down in childhood are clearer and more fixed than are the ones laid down later in life. This is why learning is easier when younger. However, nowadays, responsibility for the education of children is largely relinquished by parents and handed over to schools, television and computers. From these three major influences comes a strange and unpredictable learning experience. Most children learn by seeing the things that are repeated most often in their lives. Parents teach their children to brush their teeth every day, for example. This becomes so ingrained that, by the time we reach adulthood, we do it automatically. This is a fantastically well-taught activity, because the vital channels are clear and easily accessed. So it is with every activity that is consistent and repetitive.

Another way to create clear and well-defined vital channels is to have a dramatic learning event. When something has an emotional charge attached to it, the force of the vitality flowing through the channels makes for very speedy learning. Attaching pain to an event is one way in which the body has taken advantage of this phenomenon. Most children learn what the word 'hot' means very early on. This channel stays with you into adulthood so that, when you have a child of your own, you may be surprised by how readily you shout 'HOT!' when he or she gets close to the fire. It is not something you stop to think about.

The creation myths that we teach our children help to create our fundamental channels but not always in the ways we might expect. Children are often taught biblical stories as if they were the literal truth. Children even go along with them on one level but, on another, they know that the stories cannot be real and so they learn not to trust everything that adults say – probably a good lesson, in itself, but one which could be taught in a healthier way. The fundamental channels laid down in childhood are the ones we most easily go back to when older. This is why our childhood is so important and also why it is harder to treat anyone whose childhood contains difficult times.

Vital channels are continually created, modified and exercised from the moment we are conceived to the moment of death. Each person's channels are different. As long as there is consistency within the internal representation of the way things are, there will be full vitality and no illness is possible. As soon as inner conflict is experienced (along with its accompanying BIC) then symptoms will develop. These symptoms might be anything from a sprained ankle to liver cancer and even schizophrenia as every single illness has a distorted life force at its centre.

Creation myths

Prejudice always creates conflict.

One of the prejudices which we all hold centres around our idea of creation. The beliefs which we hold about how we are created – both individually and as a race – and what happens to us when we die have a profound effect on our feelings. This applies not only when life begins and ends but also whenever we start anything or whenever anything finishes. It happens whether we are aware of it or not.

Most of us hold more than one idea in our heads about how the universe was created, taking each on board even if they conflict with one another. If there is a conflict, we will find it difficult to create anything. This might include everything from making a meal to creating a new project to what we will do with our next holiday. Everything we create will be filtered through and influenced by these archetypal beliefs about how the world was created.

One creation myth is the belief that everything comes from Adam and Eve. This could translate into believing that the best way to create anything new is with a male/female partnership. If you were taught that the world was made in six days with a rest at the end, you may believe that it takes a week to decide or to make anything. Alternatively, you may believe that all ideas and changes come with a Big Bang, where what you want appears instantly.

It seems inevitable, then, that your views about what happens after you die also have profound effects on the way you live your life and, consequently, on your health.

The Tibetan Book of the Dead (translated by Gyurme Dorje, Penguin Classics), a book from a Tibetan Buddhist perspective, presents another creation myth. It is a description of the whole process by which you get born again into the next life, with the starting point being how you leave your last life. On the surface, it appears to contain information about the death process, but I believe another of its purposes is to inform the living how anything is created.

Understanding death

Every one of your beliefs has the potential to create conflict in you and so cause problems.

What we believe happens after we die affects us in the present. However, when you ask a person about this belief, their answer is often extremely woolly. When a person has a religious faith, they answer according to the doctrines of that faith although, very often, they do not believe it in their heart. They may not be aware that they have this conflict, yet I often see it in my practice – for example, when a Christian cannot resolve his/her grief for a loved one. They may go along with the idea of going to heaven, or hell, but when questioned a little more deeply, they say that they don't really know what happens, or that they actually think nothing happens. There are many times when the intellect will say one thing while the heart says another. That person will have inner conflict and symptoms will inevitably follow.

Yet an enlightened understanding about what happens after death is fundamental to health. This is because everyone is touched by death and most people are aware that they will die at some point. But even more importantly, our view of what happens after we die colours our view of what happens whenever anything we are involved with comes to an end. Our after-death belief will be employed in these situations also.

A full understanding of death is needed if you wish to leave behind your difficulties and become a complete, healthy human being. And yet no one knows for sure what happens after death even if they believe they do. However, if we simplify slightly, we can see that the world believes in just three possible outcomes after death.

The first possibility is annihilation, where nothing happens – just oblivion. People who have this as their main after-death belief have a very hard time, especially when someone close to them dies. They often believe that life is futile and they live for the present, knowing that when they die they will not be taking anything with them. One way forward for these people is to make their children the centre of their lives, for they can carry on their genes. If a person believes that there is nothing after death then suicide will always be an option when life gets very difficult. If this type of person does not have children, they are likely to spend a lot of time in maximizing physical pleasure, since their focus in life will be the body. The body will be all-important. They may care a lot about their own appearance and the appearance of everything else.

The second possibility is that you get reborn and go through the birth-death cycle again, commonly called re-incarnation. This is the after-death belief held by the majority of the world's people. Built into this idea is the belief that the better you are in this life, the more points you will store up, and the better and happier you will be in the next life. People who hold this belief care less about appearances but they do care about what others think of them. This shows the predominance of the ego.

The third possibility is that you get reborn in some form somewhere else and stay there forever. It may be heaven, hell or some other place. These people believe in the continuance of the Self (spirit, soul or higher self) after death.

So, essentially, there are only three possibilities concerning what happens after we die. These beliefs have their roots in the way we see ourselves as being made up of the three, discrete living-realms: *Body, Ego* and *Self.*

From the Body's point of view, when it dies there is no more. Of course, the individual cells may break down and get taken up by other life-forms but, from the Body's viewpoint, that is the end. When people perceive themselves as being only a body, they hold this belief. It is a view many people hold but you cannot always tell this from what they say. You will be able to tell through the way the person talks and acts.

From the Ego's standpoint, when it 'dies' it is instantly reborn in a never-ending cycle. You can easily experience this if you get embarrassed. The Ego even says, 'I could have died.' Actually there is a break in consciousness but the Ego immediately fills the space and is reborn.

The Self is a little different in that it just *is* and, because it is emptiness, there is nothing to die. It cannot die. It lives forever. According to St Thomas, Christ said 'the living never die', meaning that those who are truly alive have found that part of themselves which remains the same all through life. When you move your awareness into Self, you literally live forever. The only argument you will get is from your jealous Ego.

However, it is impossible to stay in one discrete living-realm for the whole of your life. As has been said, health is the ability to move freely from one to another. A healthy view of death will have to take this into account.

The truth of the matter is that all three possibilities can occur in everyone at the same time; the key to healthy living is to know this and realize that awareness can move from one discrete living-realm to another so that you do not get trapped in any particular one. People can get stuck in the Body, Ego or the Self and this is when problems arise.

Escapes

Inner conflict is difficult to live with, so why don't we try to get rid of it? The answer is that we often tend to think that the cure is worse than putting up with the symptoms. It may take only a few seconds to distract ourselves from a problem we know we have. We may do this because we know it will take a fair amount of time to actually deal with the problem completely and we tell ourselves that we don't have the time at the moment. What we don't realize is that, if we were to add up all the pain and effort we have used in distracting ourselves, it would probably be much greater than the effort required to resolve the situation. Our memories do not help in this situation. If we could reliably compare the effort involved in escaping a problem with the effort required to resolve it, we would address all of our problems. The desire to distract ourselves comes from inner conflict, which always ends in a break in consciousness. After a break in consciousness, memory is lost.

So, instead, we indulge in distractions. The tools we use to do this must be big enough to do the job. Drugs are excellent in this regard – the more powerful the drug, the more effective it will be in distracting us. They work in two ways. Their primary effect is to change your state of awareness sufficiently to allow you to forget your problem. As the primary effect wears off and the desire for the next fix becomes stronger, so nothing else matters. The drugs which fulfil this criterion are the so-called 'stimulants', such as tea, coffee, nicotine and recreational drugs such as alcohol and cannabis. Of course, illegal drugs (like heroin) also fulfil the criterion, but their use is less common because such a large distraction is only needed for people in extreme pain. The size of the distraction required exactly matches the size of the unresolved inner conflict.

Food also has a distracting power, with sugar being one of the main culprits. But everything that distracts you causes you to separate yourself from your illness, actually maintaining your inner conflict, and so to prolong it. Common culprits include shopping, TV, cinema, newspapers, and novels. These are not problems in themselves. The problem is the inner conflict; if you resolve that then the desire for distraction may well disappear.

Why do we think that the cure is worse than putting up with the symptoms? The answer is that the cure doesn't reside in the patient's own realm. It resides instead in the unknown, of which the patient is scared. It is outside their comfort zone. All escape-attempts lie inside the comfort zone. It is only when the patient lets go of what they think they know that they will get anywhere.

Different drugs allow escape in different ways. The more gentle ones, like tea and coffee, modify the current state of the person. The stronger ones always transform the current state into a familiar place regardless of the mood when the drug was taken. All drugs taken routinely are an obstacle to genuine health.

Panic attacks

As an example of thinking that the cure is worse than the symptoms, you cannot do better than to look at panic attacks.

Panic attacks are common, often mismanaged, and yet are relatively easy to resolve. A panic attack usually makes you feel that you are about to die. Imagine it: there you are minding your own business when your heart begins to pound in your body as if it were trying to escape. You break out in a cold sweat but when you look around you cannot find the source of any danger because there isn't any.

Everyone who experiences panic attacks initially tries to suppress them. So what is suppression and why is it wrong? Suppression is always caused by inner conflict, by being pulled in two different directions at the same time. The main reaction that people who experience a panic attack have is 'how do I get rid of this problem as quickly as possible?' They have a choice which they feel goes like this: which direction should I go in when every direction seems more scary than the last and staying put is terrifying? They are in a no-win situation but eventually the panic attack dies away and they can appear to get on with their life. But what has really happened? Unpleasant symptoms are generally unwanted but they are actually an attempt to resolve the problem by getting you to re-live it. This is especially true for panic attacks. They start when a traumatic experience is not resolved. This could be a physical trauma (in the case of a car accident, for instance); an emotional trauma (in the case of multiple grief) or it could be a mental trauma (as in the case of a bad drug experience). The only way to undo the symptoms is to experience fully all of the (energetic) pain of the initial experience with full awareness. As soon as a part of it is ignored or denied, that part will remain unhealed and cause problems. And when the person is in a safe place, as far as the body is concerned, and the original event is in some way stimulated, there will be an attempt to heal the situation by having the trauma replayed – a panic attack. If awareness can be brought to the whole of the panic attack, that will be the end of it – otherwise it will repeat until such time as awareness is brought to the situation.

Pills that are given to relieve the situation somehow will always fail, for the trauma is lodged energetically, internally. The *only* way to resolve it is to allow an energetic outlet for the original trauma. Of course, this can be done through a talking therapy but only if the talking therapy accesses the energy and doesn't involve suppressing the symptoms. It is far more efficient to work directly with the energy.

The externalization of inner conflict

A question arises: do *all* of our health problems stem from internal conflict, or are there external forces from which we need protection? When so much emphasis is placed on the role of vaccinations in preventing disease and of antibiotics in killing bugs, it is not surprising that bacteria and viruses are demonized. A lot of money is made out of people's fear of germs – from the cost of vaccinations to the excessive use of household cleaning products. It is acknowledged nowadays that children's immune systems are not developing well because they are not exposed to enough ordinary household germs. Even here there is conflict.

I have worked on many thousands of people who have had many different disease labels put on them and I can say that every single one of them has had a distortion in their flow of life force resulting in reduced vitality. And I also know that, if their vitality were increased, their illness would diminish. The belief that there are germs out there waiting to pounce on us is an externalization of an inner conflict. Of course, germs exist and I know that orthodox medicine attributes certain illnesses to certain bugs but, many times, you hear how even healthy people have the bug on them and yet they do not get ill.

One of the reasons that it is so easy to believe illness and disease lie outside of us and are just waiting to come and get us is that our egos cannot bear to be wrong. The reason we have a reduced or split vitality is that our ego has reduced our view of the world and we believe that we don't have enough of something. How do we get back on track? We get an illness that forces us to take stock of what we do have. The bugs that help us to do this are really only the messengers. Sometimes it feels like it helps to shoot the messenger.

And so we get ill because our ego cannot bear to be wrong (i.e. we are stuck in a realm of our own making due to an inner conflict). And there you have it; this is the very centre of my philosophy on health and disease.

Illness and disease are actually very easy to understand until you make the error of not owning your conflicts and believing that they have their roots in someone or something outside of you. Not owning conflicts has the direct result of creating many multi-billion dollar industries, one of them being the pharmaceutical industry. However, they are not evil. They are only the providers of what has been requested by orthodox medicine.

Vaccination

When we believe that the problem lies outside of ourselves, we can easily dismiss the talk about the effects that multiple vaccinations in early childhood are having on children's developing immune systems. In addition, today's children are mostly not reaping the beneficial stimulation to the immune system that the common bugs and childhood diseases gave to them in the past.

On the whole, vaccinations do what they are designed to do. They generally stop people getting some diseases. Unfortunately, that is not the whole story. If you believe, as orthodox medicine does, that disease comes from bugs, then you are doing a good job in getting people's immune system to deal with the nasties. However, a problem arises if you believe that a distorted life force due to inner conflict is at the root of all illnesses and that the bugs are there to sort out the problem. Getting rid of the symptoms is only half of the problem. It is a shame that vaccinations cannot deal with the inner conflict which creates the susceptibility to the disease.

Before there were vaccinations, people had other ways of warding off illnesses with amulets, talismans, scars and spells. It would seem that people look for external expressions of their inner split. In Jungian psychology, it is acknowledged that people are uncomfortable with their 'shadows' (the darker side of their personalities) and try to project them on to things or people outside of themselves. There, they become monsters to be feared. Only by owning our demons and working with them or with their energy can we be freed from them. Only by embracing and acknowledging both sides of the split, and then allowing the energy to move on, can we become truly whole.

All vaccination fails to address the real problem even if it appears to prevent disease.

Part 3: Disease and Becoming Healthy

What is disease?

The symptoms are not the disease. This points to a fundamental difference between western and alternative medicine. Western medicine often labels the disease according to its major symptom, which is then translated into Greek. Alternative medicine sees all of the symptoms, both major and minor, as the results of a deeper disturbance.

The word disease can refer to a specific illness, such as chicken pox or, going back to the original meaning of the word, it can mean *dis*, meaning 'opposing' or 'apart', and *ease*. Ease is not something we think about that often but it could be described as free-flowing life force. Disease is a disordered flow of life force and the symptoms which result are the consequences of that disordered life force. Because symptoms are always caused by the vitality expressing itself in the best way it can, they are neither good nor bad in themselves, even if they are unpleasant. What they do is to point to the source of the illness; in themselves, they are results, not causes. This display of symptoms is unique to each individual, even if two people have the same disease label. In western medicine, most disease labels are, in fact, just a description of the physical symptoms and are therefore not really very helpful. For example, *asthma* means 'hard breathing', *eczema* means 'boil out' and *arthritis* means 'joint inflammation'. If you went to a doctor and she diagnosed joint inflammation you may well say, 'Yes, I know that, but what is wrong with me?' and then you get a diagnosis of 'arthritis' and you say, 'Ah, I've heard of that.'

Giving the disease a name actually does very little for the patient because the name only refers to the results of the illness and not to the cause.

Most western doctors remove the body's ability to produce the symptoms it wants to because they cannot see the interconnectedness of the symptoms and the disordered life force. While removing symptoms may endear a doctor to his/her patient, if it is done without reference to the vitality of the patient then it is, at worst, irresponsible and dangerous. Why is this? Having disease labels separates the illness from the patient. The result is that the disease gets treated and the patient is forgotten. Removal of symptoms does not remove the disease; if the physician is not aware of the role of the life force in disease, it will be impossible to discover if the disease underlying the symptoms has actually gone. For example, if a person has a cold and takes something to dry up the runny nose and then goes on to develop gout, would any medical practitioner be able to see the connection? The answer is, only one who is aware of the life force. Of course, doctors and drug companies do not deliberately make people's ill-health worse. They do exactly what is asked of them – namely, they remove symptoms. Western medical doctors and drug companies do not have any reference point for the life force so they are unable to truly understand the cause of any disease.

Indeed, drug companies are often blamed for creating medicines that cause harm to people, but it is not their fault. They are simply fulfilling a role prescribed by western medicine, with scientific thinking and processes backing them up. Moreover, medical doctors are not to blame for the way in which they prescribe the drugs or for alleviating people's symptoms. They provide the service which they have been asked to provide. But this doesn't mean that things could not be better. Without understanding the role of the life force, drug companies and doctors will only be able to work on the physical level. There needs to be a radical shift in understanding by the consumer (i.e. patient) in order for things to change.

So, if the symptoms are not the disease then what is? The answer is still the same: a disordered life force brought about by inner conflict. Of course, everyone gets inner conflict; then again, everyone gets symptoms. In most cases, your inner conflicts get resolved naturally – as over time you may become a little more rational, and circumstances are always changing – and so the conflict often disappears on its own and takes with it the disordered life force. When it doesn't disappear so easily, you will get an illness like a cold which, if you are lucky, will lay you low for a few days. While you are laid low, the conflict gets resolved in a remarkable way. Whether you are aware of it or not you will be forced to 'think' about the problem. Actually, the problem doesn't exist in thoughts or even emotions: it exists in your 'energy body', in the flow of your life force. This is where your thoughts, feelings, dreams and even fantasies originate and play themselves out. In so doing, the flow of life force is re-ordered, which in turn allows you to recover. This is why dreams usually become more excited during acute illnesses.

Becoming ill

Viruses and bacteria obviously exist and play their part but they only cause a problem in people who are susceptible; this susceptibility arises solely on account of a disordered vitality. Part of the proof of this is that not everyone gets the same illnesses even if they are exposed to the same bugs.

When people fall ill, the illness they contract is not arbitrary. The symptoms are an expression of what is happening in that person's vitality. From this you may infer that you can make yourself sick and that it is your fault. In some ways you are correct, but you cannot wake up one morning and say, 'I'm going to give myself measles today.' Even so, whatever illness you have is a direct result of what has gone unresolved in your past. The cure will have to bear this in mind or you will not get better; you may even end up in a worse state.

People love to have a label for their illnesses. Giving a diagnosis appears to be the role of most medical practitioners, both orthodox and alternative. However, the disease labels that are given to collections of symptoms are of no value in any real cure, although by using the disease label and associated medication, the symptoms can often be made to disappear. For example, if someone has eczema, it is usually treated with a steroidal cream. This is a knee-jerk reaction method of prescribing. No thought is required; the patient is not taken into account; why the eczema started up is of no concern; the prescription is given according to the disease label. And on many occasions this apparently works in that the skin gets better.

The trouble with this sort of prescribing is that it generally causes problems, sometimes visible, sometimes invisible. Many times, my patients tell me that their doctor has said it is quite likely that their child with eczema will go on to develop asthma. This worsening of, and increase in, symptoms is exactly what will happen if you suppress any initial symptom. The body knows it has to express the illness and it will try to do so in the least harmful way it can. When it is denied expression through the skin, as in eczema treated with steroids, it will go to the most similar organ. In essence, the lungs are a modified version of skin in that they are in contact with the air. Asthma can be thought of as eczema on the lungs. Again, the symptom is there for a reason and, if it is suppressed through the use of steroid inhalers, there will be a more serious complication, probably with something like a severe asthma attack. Steroids can be thought of as credit card health; everything they give you has to be paid back and usually with interest.

Becoming healthy

The key to getting healthy is simple: first remove the external causes that maintain the illness and then increase the vitality. If you can understand how to do this, then I believe that every acquired illness can be cured.

The external causes that maintain illness

Toxins, dental treatment, sugar, inorganic food, medication, tea, coffee, tobacco and alcohol can all contribute to illness. Toxins to the body can include food to which you have an intolerance and the chemical additives in food. Other external causes may include background radiation, mobile phones, heavy metals and pollution. In order to become healthy all of these external causes have to be dealt with first.

Case: A patient had a problem sleeping and yet drank six mugs of coffee each day. When I asked if he knew that coffee kept people awake, he told me that he didn't have one after 5.00pm! I have personally found that one cup of coffee stops me sleeping for thirty-six hours.

Case: Another patient had a persistent cough. She eventually admitted that she smoked twenty cigarettes each day; when she stopped her cough disappeared.

Tea often causes headaches. I would be surprised if anyone could drink six or more mugs of tea per day without feeling its effects. Alcohol can make people irritable long before it becomes addictive. Sugar, although it initially gives energy, goes on to rob you of energy. Most prescribed medication is unnecessary and is only given to suppress symptoms. Nowadays, a lot of people are sensitive to dairy, wheat or some other modified food stuff. Mobile telephones cause both me and my wife a problem with our ears, so how can they not cause others a problem? It all adds up to a host of problems that, luckily, can be solved fairly easily. Indeed, the majority of people's ailments would disappear if they just looked at their relationship with the substances mentioned here. Food additives and colourings can also cause many problems – mental, emotional and physical.

Case: A seven-year-old girl had been labelled 'hyperactive' by her teacher, who also suggested putting her on Ritalin. Before taking this step, her parents wanted to see if anything else could help her. On questioning her mother about her diet and what she drank, it was discovered that she was drinking an ordinary sugar-free squash on a daily basis. On putting my hands on her head and 'tuning in', I could feel that the artificial sweetener in the squash was doing strange things to the energy flowing through her head, scattering her thinking processes and making it very hard for her to sustain any concentration. On my advice, she stopped drinking anything with artificial sweeteners and her behaviour returned to normal. The teachers said that her change in behaviour in the classroom was remarkable. She did not need further treatment.

Case: A thirteen-year-old boy had been diagnosed with ADHD and had been taking Ritalin for six years. He was sensitive to a few different foods and chemical additives, but the substance that was giving him the most problems was wheat. He had an addictive relationship with wheat, in which he ate nothing that did not contain wheat, as he knew it would not satisfy his craving. The effect that wheat was having on him was like a toxic drug: he craved it and suffered from withdrawal when he came off it. His behaviour calmed down considerably just by giving up wheat, and many unwanted physical symptoms, such as chronic constipation, also disappeared. It took him a few weeks to get used to not being 'drugged up' by the wheat and adjust to what he described as 'feeling normal' and 'thinking more clearly'. He also needed three sessions of the Boulderstone Technique to resolve the birth trauma he had suffered, which had contributed to his behavioural problems. His behaviour and moods improved greatly and he was able to come off the Ritalin that he had been on since the age of seven.

The internal causes that maintain illness

Lack of forgiveness.

Illness can be maintained mentally and emotionally. A major cause of maintaining illness is the inability to forgive someone for hurting you. Many people think that they are due an apology for a hurt which they have experienced but this is always a mistake and will inevitably lead to some form of illness. Someone once said that not forgiving a person was similar to taking poison and expecting the other person to die from it. You hurt yourself by not forgiving but it may feel like you are handing out justice to someone who has hurt you.

Most people, when confronted by their non-forgiving attitude and the consequences of it, say that they know it is causing them a problem. I know a woman who is aggressive towards men but relates well to women. A man must have hurt her sometime in the past because her excuse is, 'Oh, I have a problem with men,' as if that is some kind of answer. This woman has been saying this for over ten years and she is still not prepared to forgive. Holding on to problems can seem a comfortable option if you are not aware of their wider implications.

Forgiveness is often held back because it is felt that if you forgive it will mean that the 'perpetrator' will get away without punishment. Somehow, in the mind of the hurt person, not forgiving is meant to punish the person who has done the hurting. But this is another mistaken belief. Who does forgiving really affect? The person who has done the hurting may not even be aware that they have been forgiven. The person forgiving has to go through a process of truly understanding the bigger picture, the context of the perceived hurt. If they can go through this process, see the bigger picture and forgive, then they will come out without baggage. Otherwise they could carry the hurt around with them for the rest of their life. So should you forgive everybody? The point is that judgement creates for you a realm in which you are acting like a god. Whilst inside this realm everything is rosy, but this realm will conflict with your other realms, inner conflict will follow and so, eventually, will physical symptoms. Forgiveness is the only solution.

A father killed himself on his daughter's birthday. It took over twenty years for the daughter to finally forgive her father, and the symptoms of overeating, betrayal of friendships, pathological lying and other attempts to distract herself from her pain slowly came to an end. Whenever a hurt is the cause of symptoms, forgiveness is the best step forward. Two good books on the subject are *The Journey* by Brandon Bays (HarperCollins, 1999) and *Core Transformation* by Connirae and Tamara Andreas (Real People Press, 1996). The ultimate book on forgiveness is *A Course in Miracles* (Foundation for Inner Peace, 2001).

Allopathic medicine and symptom removal

Allopathic medicine is used both in acute and chronic conditions. Its purpose is to modify the condition of the patient and, in this respect, it usually has an effect. If it didn't, it wouldn't be used. However, except in special circumstances, even though it may remove the symptoms, it also reduces the vitality of the patient. Symptom removal may indeed be exactly what the patient is after but that is because the patient has grown up in a world where the connection between vitality and symptoms is not understood.

A lot of allopathic medicines are symptom-removal drugs. They are the 'anti' drugs – such as anti-inflammatories, anti-depressants, antibiotics, painkillers, anti-histamines and the most important of the 'anti' drugs: steroids, which are basically 'anti-symptoms'. All of these drugs aim to remove symptoms without recognizing their cause. From a health point of view, they are bad news. Although they actually do their job (in that the *symptoms* often do disappear). The *disease* often stays in place, continuing to develop and grow until it manifests in a bigger and more complex health problem. The problem here is that the philosophy (i.e. symptom removal) does not provide a cure. Unfortunately, orthodox medicine will not be able to see the cause of illness until it recognizes the existence of the life force. It can neither effect a cure intentionally nor recognize true cure, as it doesn't adhere to a philosophy, or follow a methodology, that operates from a concept of true health.

Allopathy doesn't even cure when surgery is employed, as the energetic cause of the problem is still not addressed. Surgery is usually a last resort and, again, it is an attempt simply to remove the symptom without giving much regard to the cause of the problem. Certainly, an alcoholic who needs a liver transplant will be told to stop drinking but his reasons for drinking will not be examined – certainly not by the surgeon, anyway. For all their skill, surgeons are really only mechanics. Real health practice is actually carried out after the operation by the patient as he/she comes to terms with what has happened, supported by caring nurses and family, if they are lucky. Or, more likely, they carry on as before, leaving the real disease in place.

And yet many people do get better after seeing a western medical practitioner. This is usually because the patient is given a temporary boost of vitality – possibly as the result of having their problem focused on and taken seriously, or simply through the healing interaction between doctor and patient. This healing interaction has been labelled the placebo effect and, because it is not easily reproduced, is often dismissed as irrational, immeasurable and, therefore, unscientific.

Increasing vitality

If western medicine does not address the vitality, what does? There are many methods of increasing your vitality but they all amount to the same thing: removing the 'breaks in consciousness' and healing the inner conflicts which cause them. The most efficient method of doing this is probably the Boulderstone Technique of Life Force Healing because it addresses these problems directly. (Why this is so will be described in depth later.) Really facing up to a problem is a way of increasing vitality. This may be a doctor's greatest gift. For example, diagnosis of a life-threatening disease can bring anyone face to face with their own mortality and may force an honest review of the sufferer's lifestyle, in turn allowing changes to be made more easily. If someone is aware of your deepest fear and can stand alongside you at this time, it can give you the strength and vitality to move on from this place. This is what a good doctor, homeopath or any other health professional can do. Even when it is called the placebo effect, if its power is underestimated something important will be lost. There are many other ways to increase vitality – including exercise, meditation, martial arts, listening to music and viewing art. The list is virtually endless.

Why people sometimes give up on a true healing programme

As you increase your vitality, so your problems become more accessible and are therefore more easily removed. You get the energy to deal with the problem. However, because they are more obvious to you, it can feel as though your symptoms are getting worse or that there are more of them. At this point, unless you understand this process, you may give up your improvement strategy and resort to previous strategies which do not cure but may well palliate. This path will, of course, maintain the illness.

Symptoms and health

Do all symptoms disappear when you are healthy? What use is a cure if there are still symptoms left? After losing a limb, can a person ever be healthy again? Of course they can; they can even be healthier! It is not the objective symptoms that determine the health of a person. I have said many times that illness comes about through inner conflict and that this is what needs to be addressed before the patient can become truly healthy.

After successful treatment of serious debilitating diseases, such as Multiple Sclerosis, some people will recover completely in the eyes of the world while some will not. However, if cure occurs, any symptoms left over will not matter to the patient. Their inner pain and conflict will be over, they will feel at peace within – this is the primary goal.

Case 1: A woman in her seventies with terminal pancreatic cancer came for treatment using the Boulderstone Technique. The tumour was palpable energetically but not easily removed. Whilst working on the distortion in the life force, what emerged was that this woman had been carrying deep-seated emotional trauma from childhood which she had never been able to resolve. Through a combination of talking about it and restoring the flow of life force energetically, she was able to reach a point of complete peace. She felt that all her past hurts had been healed and her mind had a clarity which she had never experienced before. The healing was complete but it did not artificially keep her alive. She felt that her time had come and was ready to die peacefully from the growing tumour, a few months later. She died free of inner conflicts.

Case 2: This is a woman in her fifties, with Multiple Sclerosis going back at least twenty-five years. She has been wheelchair-bound for many years and recently had a relapse (which caused incontinence) and is slowly losing the use of her right arm. After a few months of treatment, working on herself and coming for an hour every week, she has regained bladder control and no longer has any problems with either of her arms. She does not expect to regain the use of her legs since they have deteriorated too much over the years. However, she is overjoyed at what the treatment has done for her. 'Life Force Healing has given me my life back. I had lost all enthusiasm for living and now I don't worry about things that don't need to be worried about. Now my love of life is back and I realize that life is far from over, even though I need the wheelchair to go anywhere. I have more energy than I've had in years and I feel more in control of my M.S. I know I won't get any worse now.'

Cure is always possible but it only occurs when the disordered vital force, caused by inner conflict, is restored to its clear, natural state. Then the patient will recognize that they have been healed, typically using phrases such as, 'I feel so much better in myself' and 'I have more energy than I have ever had'. The fact that they still get the odd symptom of illness does not detract from this basic step-up in vitality.

Even when cure occurs, in some cases the patient is not aware of what has contributed to the healing. Variations on the following conversations have happened many times with patients. These are typical responses from people with any long-term condition.

Case 1:
Practitioner: Did the healing help you?
Patient: No, not really. I didn't feel much happening.
Practitioner: Did your symptoms improve?
Patient: Yes, they did, but they were getting better anyway.
Practitioner: But you had the problem for seven years and you were getting worse by the year.
Patient: I suppose that's true ...

Case 2:
Practitioner: Did the Boulderstone Technique help you?
Patient: It's difficult to tell.
Practitioner: Why is that?
Patient: My symptoms haven't gone.
Practitioner: Do they bother you now?
Patient: No, I've accepted them.
Practitioner: When you first came here you were in despair about your symptoms, your relapses were happening once or twice a year and you were on steroids a lot of the time. Now you don't have any relapses and you are much happier. How do you explain this?
Patient: I've sorted myself out. I just had to.
Practitioner: Do you still do the exercises you were shown?
Patient: Oh, yes.
Practitioner: Do they help?
Patient: I'm not sure.
Practitioner: So why do you do them?
Patient: I haven't anything else to do.

Illness creeps up on people and when true healing occurs, so does cure. I quite often hear the phrase, 'I was getting better anyway' but I know it isn't true. I think people say it because, with life force therapies, they do not experience any drug-like effects and the cure can be gentle and subtle in its action. Also, when a symptom simply disappears, people have an amazing capacity to forget that they ever had it. Even so, sometimes people experience a dramatic improvement and are very clear that the treatment has helped. However, when they experience a similar problem again in the future, they forget about coming to see me and instead go to see an orthodox practitioner who often makes them worse. This leads me to believe that people quite like the cure to be painful.

I have also noticed that, as people get better, the way in which they describe how they are changes. Someone who has to lie down in a darkened room with a migraine may say that they are OK but just want to be left alone. The next day, when the migraine has gone, they may complain at length about the pressure they are under, although they are no longer in pain. Once the overwhelming symptom (such as head pain) has gone, the underlying causes often present themselves for attention. Symptom-description is a complicated business. In many cases, people tell you their symptoms but they don't tell you what's wrong. As a healer you need to address what is wrong.

How to recover from acute and chronic illness

According to homeopathic philosophy, an acute illness is one that ends in recovery or death! Generally, most people are a little too quick to take any medicine and, since the vast majority of acute illnesses end in complete recovery anyway, taking any medication will probably just add confusion to the life force. It is generally better to let the body heal itself without intervention from therapy or medication.

However, if the distorted life force can be contacted and allowed to change until it flows smoothly again, the illness will begin to resolve itself. This contact can be achieved in many different ways.

The more direct the contact, regardless of the therapy, the more efficient the process. Even though the therapy is an important consideration, the therapist is possibly even more important. An enlightened surgeon may be better able to help than will a mechanically-minded homeopath who prescribes according to disease labels.

Nowadays, there are many therapies available – which ones increase the vitality most effectively? At the top of the list are those which affect the vital force most directly: acupuncture, homeopathy and other forms of life force healing. However, even with these therapies, if the therapist cannot get their own prejudices out of the way in order to see the patient clearly, they will not be able to facilitate a cure.

Recovering from a chronic illness is no different from recovering from an acute one, except that the former is a very difficult thing for a human being to contend with. Drugs have their place (usually to relieve symptoms) but, in the long term, they slow down cure. The only way to cure is to address the underlying problem of life force disturbance. There are many things that can help this process, although most of them are not obvious. The first to look at is pain.

Pain

Pain can be crippling but, like a lot of things in life, there are two sides to it. The not-so-obvious side is that pain can be an asset – but only if you know how to deal with it. Pain can be divided into many different categories but, to begin with, I want to divide it into just two: *active pain* and *remembered pain*. *Active pain* is pain that results from something that is happening in the present. For example, if you place your hand in a flame, you will burn it and, while that is happening and while the tissues are hot, it will be painful. *Remembered pain* is a memory (though it can feel like active pain) of a painful event which is difficult or uncomfortable for you to remember – you may shut your eyes and wince while recalling it. I am sure that most people can remember a situation which they want to forget and which has this wincing quality to it. Unfortunately, these two very different feelings often get confused – a situation which is not helped by their sharing a name: pain.

Active pain exists in order to get you to move away quickly from whatever is causing the problem, to prevent further damage. The second sort of pain, remembered pain, exists because you were not fully present when you first experienced the difficult event in question. Your body/mind will keep returning to the memory of the event so that you can bring your presence to it; only fully experiencing the event will allow you to live without the wincing quality. History, and the event, do not change but your reaction to them can, turning the wince into just a memory. When full consciousness is present, pain is impossible: instead, there is sensation. Sensation becomes pain when awareness is withdrawn.

When confronted with remembered pain, you have two choices: you can move away from it, or you can move towards it and go through it, as in the nursery rhyme, 'The Bear Hunt'. Unfortunately, unless you have learned otherwise, the tendency is to move away from it. This will maintain the pain. If you move towards remembered pain, and do so with awareness, it turns that

---

The Bear Hunt

We're going on a bear hunt,
We're going to catch a big one
I'm not scared,
What a beautiful day,
Oh oh, grass,
Long wavy grass,
We can't go over it,
We can't go under it,
We'll have to go through it...
We're going on a bear hunt,
We're going to catch a big one
I'm not scared,
What a beautiful day,
Oh oh, mud,
Thick squelchy mud,
We can't go over it,
We can't go under it,
We'll have to go through it...

We're going on a bear hunt,
We're going to catch a big one
I'm not scared,
What a beautiful day,
Oh oh, a cave,
A dark gloomy cave,
We can't go over it,
We can't go under it,
We'll have to go through it...
We're going on a bear hunt,
We're going to catch a big one
I'm not scared,
What a beautiful day,
Oh oh, one wet shiny nose
Two sharp pointed teeth,
Two long furry ears,
What do you think it is?
A Bear

remembered pain into sensation. A new vital path is laid down; the next time you traverse that path, you can view the whole thing with awareness. It is always easier to travel a path that has already been traversed and so the remembered pain will be gone for good. Advanced yoga practitioners are usually aware of the difference between active pain and remembered pain. In contrast, dancers and athletes are often trained to ignore their body's warning signals and push beyond the pain barrier. While they can all become very flexible, the dancers and athletes are more likely to injure themselves on the way.

The end of the path of experiencing remembered pain is cure, free from trouble and all other difficulties. In fact, pain symptoms are largely forgotten. They can be remembered but only in the abstract; when we remember healed pain, we do not get the physical experience of it. The Chinese have a saying: 'when the shoe fits, the foot is forgotten.' This is the 'forgetting' that happens at the end of the path when awareness is maintained. Traversing the path may be difficult emotionally and mentally and sometimes it can even be scary. In many cases, this is the reason people try to avoid the journey and so are condemned to maintain their remembered pain. The problem is that maintaining remembered pain results in more symptoms because you are telling yourself, 'It's OK to have this inner conflict. I will just grow with it.'

Western medicine or an alternative?

Of all the therapies available, how can you tell which one is the most effective in any given situation? I stumbled upon how to answer this question while reading about the controversy between Louis Pasteur and Antoine Bechamp. Pasteur is considered to be one of the most important figures in the development of vaccination, but Bechamp claimed that Pasteur stole his ideas AND got them wrong by oversimplifying them. As we understand it nowadays, and as a method of wiping out a disease, vaccination certainly seems to work in general (if not in every case). So where is the problem? The problem, as always, arises because vaccination does not take vitality into consideration. What if vaccinating a person prevents them from getting the disease? Isn't that a good thing? It is certainly not a good thing that people die from preventable diseases, but disease does not start with a bug. This western medical idea is an oversimplification. What actually happens is that the person about to get ill has developed a susceptibility brought about by withdrawing awareness. Ideally, the body would address this susceptibility before getting ill, but it doesn't know how. While the body is trying to work out how to resolve the problem, the withdrawn awareness means that it doesn't notice when a bug enters its system. And so symptoms develop.

I have worked with many different therapists and I believe that each therapy works within its own field of reference. The problems begin when you compare any energetic therapy with western medicine. Because western medicine doesn't understand the value of vitality, it is unable to see the whole picture and, as a result, it often ridicules alternative therapies. Yet alternative therapies still thrive. For example, I have often heard it said that a homeopathic remedy cannot work as it contains no molecules of an 'active' substance. While this may be true from the point of view of medical science, from an energetic point of view it always has an effect. This may not always be discernible by the patient (if it is the wrong remedy for them at the time); nonetheless, it always has an effect. Using my awareness of the life force, I can feel the effect that a homeopathic remedy has on a patient. This is a subtler and more accurate way of assessing what effect energy medicine has on the body. The classic double-blind trials used to test some (but certainly not all) allopathic medicines are largely inappropriate for testing the efficacy of alternative therapies.

Furthermore, animal experiments are unnecessary and will not develop any cure. All they can do is show which drugs suppress which symptoms. Without an awareness of the part vitality plays in health and disease, this kind of medical research will continue to waste time and money as well as causing the unnecessary suffering of animals.

Phantom limb pain

After developing the Boulderstone Technique of Life Force Healing, I realized that it was a therapy which could help many people with problems that were just not being addressed by western medicine. One of the first problems I focused on was phantom limb pain. Phantom pain is always remembered pain. In many cases, especially with traumatic injuries, there is a very large wincing factor, indicating that the patient wants to move away from the problem. This distraction actually holds the pain in place; the only way to clear the pain is to 'go through it'. After amputation, as many as 80% of people feel pain in their non-existent limb. The problem, of course, is a distorted flow of life force – caused either by a disease process or accident or by the amputation itself. Either way, phantom limb pain is a relatively easy problem to sort out with the therapy I have developed. However, in the UK at least, no one working with the problem has so far shown much interest. The health professionals whom I encountered in the USA were a little more open-minded and I was able to help more amputees with this problem. There may be many reasons for this resistance to an alternative solution, but one of the most significant, I think, is that western medicine is still generally considered to be the one valid therapy, even when it fails to find a solution. What is more, in the UK at least, there is a widespread illusion that proper medical care is free; anyone who charges for their services is viewed with suspicion. In the USA, people are generally more aware of the cost of allopathic medicine and are in a better position to judge value for money.

Parts of the body can only regenerate if the life force is still flowing. I have worked with many people who have lost a limb in traumatic circumstances. In many cases, I can feel that the life force is still disturbed – even many years after the original accident. In these cases, phantom limb pain is always present. Using my own life force, it is possible to straighten out the distortions and remove the phantom limb pain. However, the limb will not grow back. It may try to and the stump may produce growth spurs but, if too much tissue is removed, no regeneration is possible. I do not know whether the work on stem cells will make limb regeneration possible but I suspect that, if it were ever to happen, unless the distortion in the life force is corrected, the new growth will also be distorted.

Symptoms / diseases

The symptoms of an illness are not the disease:
they are the pointers back to health.

Generally, most people with chronic illnesses say that they want to get better. Even so, they are often (albeit unwittingly) actually holding the illness and symptoms in place. Tibetan medicine says that all illness comes from ignorance; this is also my understanding. Nobody wants difficult symptoms – everyone wants to be symptom-free and happy – but if what you have done and are still doing causes you to be ill, why don't you look for a solution elsewhere? The answer is that you may not be aware that there are alternatives – such is the grip that western medicine has on our health. Another reason why you might not look for a solution is that you believe you know what the solution is but think it would be too difficult to implement. For example, you know alcohol is bad for you but you still drink on a regular basis and feel sick. Giving up appears to be harder than not giving up. This all changes when you start to address the impaired flow of life force. As you become more aware of your inner vitality, the craving for external stimulants diminishes and you start to make healthier choices which increase your energy rather than diminish it.

Physical problems

How you create illness.

When I was fourteen, I used to pretend that I had a stomach ache in order to avoid school. It sometimes worked and my mother would let me stay at home. Looking back on this time in my life, I can see some things which I was not able to see at the time. The first is that, as a fourteen-year-old, I felt it was a difficult time for me. In retrospect, it was not particularly hard (in fact, it was fairly easy) – I just didn't like school. I was reasonable at some subjects but I considered a lot of what I did to be a waste of time. On one level, the pain I pretended to have was not real. On another level, I did have emotional pain that I did not know how to express. I also think that I would have been ignored if I had tried to express it. I invented a stomach ache to take away the emotional pain of having to go to school. Somehow, subconsciously, I related the stomach ache to the emotional pain I was experiencing in going to school and it worked: as a result of my pretence, I had less emotional pain because I avoided going to school. This is what your body does, too: for every mental and emotional problem you have, there is a related physical part that will eventually develop a corresponding problem.

This does not mean that an emotional problem creates a physical problem. Rather, the difficulty which lies behind them both creates both. This difficulty is always created by an inner conflict. Inner conflicts lie behind feelings, thoughts and physical sensations. See if you can feel one inside you now. The place where it exists is what I am calling your 'energetic body', your vitality. However, without always being aware of it, we are always connected to our energetic body. This point is important because it may suggest that you can affect the flow of life force using thoughts and feelings, but this is not the case. Thoughts and feelings follow the life force. When you practise life force healing on someone, you are manipulating the life force directly. The resulting restoration of the flow of energy then has a powerful transformative effect on thoughts and feelings, as well as on the physical body.

Thoughts and feelings are very closely associated with the flow of energy but, as you work with them, you begin to see that they operate in different ways. Thoughts are rational and feelings are non-rational. People tend to let either thoughts or feelings dominate most aspects of their life. Stereotypically, men work with thoughts and women with feelings but, in reality, both are working with the underlying flow of life force which is expressed *through* thoughts and feelings. If a person is following their flow of life force and it is expressed through their thoughts, they may well make giant leaps in understanding yet not know how they got there. This is where intuition comes from.

Accidents

During a physical accident, pain arises which often overwhelms a person. This feeling of being overwhelmed is where problems arise, and where inner conflict comes from. If total awareness can be kept while the pain is being experienced, no residual problem will remain. However, when you withdraw awareness because the problem is too difficult to hold in your consciousness, you are saying to your body, 'I promise I'll deal with this hard bit later.' All your problems in life must be dealt with but some of them can be put off for a while. This ability to put off solving problems is what separates human beings from all other animals and is also the reason why other animals do not suffer the range of illnesses that we do. In humans, a large number of chronic diseases and mental illnesses result from not dealing with issues soon after they arise, but allowing them to fester.

The notion of withdrawing awareness in order to deal with the difficult problem at a later date arises from the belief that you cannot deal with it at the time. This, then, causes the inner conflict which is the core of all illness, both physical and mental. It arises because we do not understand the two different kinds of pain.

During an accident, awareness may be partly removed (fully removing it would mean becoming unconscious or fainting) but, on an unconscious level, everything is experienced and nothing is forgotten. Unless the difficulty of this experience is resolved soon after, the mind and/or body will start to make a 'fuss'. This indicates where attention is needed to bring about recovery from the accident. The 'fuss' that it makes is similar to the manner in which the original accident is remembered by the body. It is stored in an energetic form and thus can have an effect on the body, thinking mind and emotions. If painkillers are taken, as they often are, the unresolved part goes into hiding for a while, regroups and then tries to find another way of expressing itself. Although this is an energetic process, it will also be experienced physically, mentally and/or emotionally until the healing is complete.

This whole process is, in fact, a universal law and one over which no negotiation is possible. It is true for all accidents, not just physical ones. Emotional 'accidents', such as the sudden death of a parent or spouse, follow the same laws. The 'law' states that *everything that happens to you must be dealt with or it will have consequences*.

Sometimes things happen which are impossible for us to understand or to deal with properly at the time. This is especially true of children and is the reason they need to be protected from trauma which they are ill-equipped to handle. When they do experience traumatic events, the adults around them can help a great deal by going through the event and allowing the child to relive all the feelings associated with their experience. It is particularly helpful to encourage them to cry and also to shake as much as they need to in order to discharge their shock and fear. Holding shock or other emotions in the vitality will cause problems later on.

All overwhelming accidents or traumas which are not dealt with completely are stored. However, they are stored not in the physical body but in the vitality, which informs the body how to be and grow. It is the storing of trauma that gives rise to the disordered flow of life force which, in turn, gives rise to distorted vitality and illness. The good news is that all stored trauma can be eliminated; a life force healer knows how to do this.

A case of whiplash

A woman who had had a whiplash injury for two years came to see me. In that time she had seen her doctor who had referred her to an orthopaedic surgeon. He, in turn, told her to see a physiotherapist, which she then did, but her neck got no better. In fact, it soon started to affect her whole life. She went to see chiropractors and cranial osteopaths, but all to no avail. Finally, she came to see me. The person who recommended me to her had told her that I was a healer, but both she and her family thought that healers were all charlatans. However, by this stage she was fairly desperate and so she allowed me to treat her using the Boulderstone

Technique. It is a simple matter to undo the effects of whiplash. With my hands on her head, I followed the twists and turns in which her head wanted to move, re-visiting what had happened to her body during the accident. All the contorted movements, and also the shock, were stored like a memory blueprint in her life force and she only needed a little help to release these energetic patterns through movement. When I had finished, she got up and said it felt a bit better. I heard later that it had completely cured her, that her operation was cancelled and she went about her life. I have never heard from her again and I am told that she will not tell even her own family that it was a healer who helped her.

Arthritis

The physical body follows the flow of life force. This can be clearly seen when the life force distorts the fingers of the hand, as in the case of arthritis.

A person's hands do not get distorted like this without strong forces being constantly applied to them. If your hands are healthy, try now to distort your fingers so that they mimic the shape of those in the picture. It requires huge force.

I can feel these forces in people who have arthritic hands but I can also feel these forces in people who do not yet have arthritic hands. I believe that they would go on to develop distorted hands if the restrictions in their life force were not removed. In fact, I have seen many people in every decade of their life, from the teens onwards, who have pains and swellings in the joints of their fingers. I soon realized that their life force was pulling their fingers sideways from the second and third knuckle in a direction away

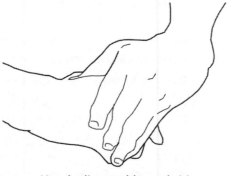

Hands distorted by arthritis

from their body. I knew that, if this was allowed to continue, these hands would become deformed. I treated them and they do not now have a problem.

In each case, the fingers were subjected to forces that were greater than the muscles could cope with. This had come about because the patients were lifting things using the sides of their fingers. In one particular case, a man was rowing without having his fingers in line with his arm. The resulting unresolved strain was being stored in the energetic body and not released. This was because, in order to do so, the fingers would have had to move into a 'remembered pain' position and, since the people concerned could not tell the difference between remembered and actual pain, the 'strain' stayed in position. And so, without life force healing, the distortion remains unresolved. As the body naturally replaces its cells, it does so according to the layout of the life force, and so the deformity pictured opposite develops.

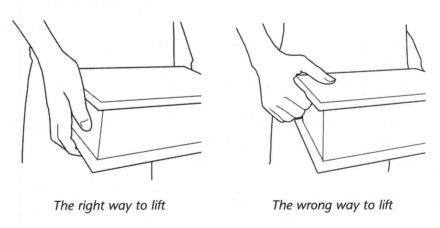

The right way to lift   The wrong way to lift

A Case of Dupuytrens

A woman in her fifties, who had had Dupuytrens Contracture for several years, came for treatment. The fingers of her right hand were noticeably distorted. Working on her right hand, I could feel how the energy flow was cramped up and twisted, giving rise to the physical distortion. The energy flow was, in fact, irregular all the way up her arm, and needed help in straightening out. After one session, she reported that her hand felt much more comfortable and less stiff and that she was able to use all of her fingers properly when driving and carrying bags. After the second session, the energy was flowing freely and there were no more symptoms of Dupuytrens. I was also able to check the left hand and both feet and confirm that similar symptoms were not likely to develop there, as the energy was flowing normally. In this way, the Boulderstone Technique can be used to check for the very earliest signs of potential symptoms before they start to show in the physical body.

How the body changes

The unresolved forces which cause problems are, in fact, replicated by the way in which our body grows and learns. The pattern of flow of the life force informs the body how to grow and how to function. To build muscles, you exercise them until you feel that they cannot do any more, then you push yourself to do more. This creates an unresolved force; the body uses this information to grow more muscle. It is the same with memory. If you consistently try to remember the maximum you can, your memory will improve. Make any effort and the body uses the information to learn to improve – it thinks that you are going to repeat what you have done and it wants to be better prepared next time.

However, if you use your body in a way with which it cannot naturally cope (such as lifting with your fingers sideways) then it will grow in such a way as to enable it to cope better – hence the distorted fingers. Right principle, wrong direction. These are rules and restrictions which you ignore at your peril.

The healing method

You can always make yourself more sensitive.

It is possible to make yourself sensitive to the movement of life force. For example, if someone came to me with a strained finger, I would hold the finger and feel the pull of the life force in the same direction in which the finger was strained. I would then allow the finger to move in the way it wanted to, although this can sometimes be painful. However, the pain is always bearable because it is remembered pain. When the finger reaches the endpoint of its movement, the body brings the life force and the finger back to a resolved position. This can take anything from ten seconds to twenty minutes or longer. When this has happened, the problem is over – no more strain and no arthritis in years to come. The 'healing' does not need to be repeated unless the person is continually injuring the part without knowing it. There is no more pain or swelling. What could be simpler?

I suspect that every case of osteo-arthritis has a strain injury at its root. I have worked on ankles that were chronically weak ever since being sprained ten years prior to the patient's coming to see me, and have seen the problem resolve inside twenty minutes. The ankle, or whatever the joint may be, gains integrity as the life force flows through it evenly. The patient also knows that the problem is resolved. Sometimes they may say that they do not believe it but inside they know. Most often they just say, 'That's amazing!'

The life force flow can also get distorted while growing, and as a result of certain enduring diseases. When it does get distorted, growing pains develop and a condition such as Osgood Schlatters can result. Actually, this is just a fancy name for growing pains, which can be effectively resolved using the Boulderstone Technique.

If you can feel the distorted flow of life force in another person and be aware of how this relates to their illness, you will know how disease and illness work and so be able to cure them.

Stress

Stress is another word for inner conflict. It causes you to be aware of your weak points and can therefore be useful. When you are feeling stressed, it is a good time to look at what is going on inside your head. Are there two conflicting thoughts or emotions present, or some other conflict in your life which you need to sort out? It is amazing how stress can just melt away when inner conflicts are resolved.

Tumours and cancer

Every tumour will have a lie at its centre.

The physical body only knows what to do because it follows the flow of life force. This can be felt by life force healers. When the life force flows back on itself and creates a loop, this loop provides the possibility for the body to grow a tumour. This energetic loop can happen when someone persists in believing something that part of them knows is not true. They continue to nurse this belief in the face of all evidence to the contrary or even their own conscience. The life force cannot flow smoothly at this point but goes around the stubborn thought or belief, which almost starts to take on a life of its own because it is at odds with the surrounding reality.

Disease occurs first in the flow of life force, and is created by our unwillingness to deal with a situation. Once the distortion exists, it will be perceived by every cell but only expressed in the way that is the most direct and that will do the least harm. Symptoms only get worse as the distortion in the life force becomes more entrenched; many opportunities arise for the resolution of the distortion. You have to fight to avoid getting better, but many people do just that because they do not understand the true nature of symptoms.

For example, after the tsunami in the Indian Ocean in 2004, I met many people in Sri Lanka who were deeply affected by this disaster. Even months afterwards, every person I met would still be relating their story. This is a natural reaction to such a disaster and a way in which people can undo the distortion in their own life force. However, I met one person who kept repeating the same story and couldn't get out of this repetitive loop. This loop, although expressed as speech, actually existed as an energetic distortion. I believe that the person in question will have many opportunities to break free of the loop in the future – not least because people will get bored of hearing the same story over and over and will eventually say as much to her. If she has enough spare energy for self-reflection, she may see what she is doing, otherwise the energetic loop will become so entrenched that I believe that her physical body will grow its own 'loop' – or, in other words, a tumour. The only solution is to address the life force distortion. Surgery that removes a tumour but leaves the original distortion in place will probably just produce another tumour unless the organ itself is removed. In that case, the loop will be expressed by the next most suitable part of the body, such as another organ. For example, removing the breasts will not truly cure breast cancer but will make it impossible for the body to express the underlying cancer in its chosen way. If the underlying energetic disease is not cured, physiological cancer may well re-appear in a deeper part of the body, such as the ovaries, lungs or bones.

Malignant tumours
A lie with attitude.

Western medicine forces the patient to view only the physical aspect of disease.

I believe that cancer, as with all illness, can *only* be cured energetically. Of course, that *can* happen within the orthodox field but it doesn't happen by design. What actually happens is that, when death approaches, the important things in life become more obvious. Keeping up a front (a possible cause for the illness in that it fosters inner conflict) can lose its value which, in turn, can allow true healing to occur.

When energy flows back on itself and a loop is created, a growth will physically develop. When the loop contains some strongly conflicting feelings, a malignant tumour may grow. For example, if someone experiences bereavement and refuses to look at the situation, an energetic loop may well be formed. If the person they lost died in such a way that it was difficult to look back at the death, within the loop could also be a focus for intolerable inner conflict. This is the kind of situation in which a malignant growth may occur.

Case: A man in his seventies presented with cancer of the oesophagus, diagnosed two months previously. He believed that he had actually had it for two years, because at that time he started suffering from heartburn for the first time in his life. His doctor prescribed an antacid which he had now been taking for two years, while his symptoms continued to get worse. Four years previously, his brother had died from a cancer that had started in exactly the same place. The patient was shattered when his brother died and was aware that his health went into decline from that point onwards. I noticed that he played with his throat when he talked about his brother. After treatment to restore the flow of his life force, the patient was able to stop the antacid without being troubled by any more heartburn or any of the other symptoms that had been building up. He felt a definite increase in his energy and his sense of wellbeing and general comfort. He slept better than previously and felt generally better and better with each treatment. He also talked about his brother a great deal and felt that he was finally working through his grief. He was very much in two minds about going ahead with the surgery, but decided he would. Sadly, his vitality was knocked so much by the operation that he came down with one health problem after another and finally died three months later of pneumonia. Needless to say, the surgeons were satisfied that the operation to remove the tumour had been a complete success. It was smaller than they had thought and the area around it was completely clear of cancer cells.

Infections, colds and flu

Every illness is unique and each person will display their illness differently even if they share the same label. Western medicine tends to group diseases together but this grouping is not useful in leading to a cure. For example, if you have a cold you could get a blocked nose or a streaming nose or both; you could feel hot, feel cold or both; you could feel sad or emotionally better than normal. Mentally, you could feel clear or foggy. You may have a headache, backache, or aching joints; your eyes may run, and so on. Every 'cold' is different. In addition to the fact that a single disease-name produces different symptoms, there is often no clear dividing line between differently-named illnesses – colds run into flu, bronchitis, pneumonia and coughs. For homeopaths, and some other alternative practitioners, the name of the disease and the diagnosis (concerned with determining whether a bacteria or a virus is involved) are not relevant. Homeopaths prescribe a remedy according to the symptom picture alone, not according to the disease label.

What determines which illness a person may succumb to? The answer is, the ill person him/herself. Everyone has their weak points which are unique to that individual. Personally, I can tell when a cold is coming on because I often get a distinctive taste in my mouth. Most people, in fact, get an indication that they have a cold coming on with a distinctive symptom unique to each individual. Some people, when they are stressed, develop a cold, flu, bronchitis, a cold sore, and so on. Others may develop a skin rash, eczema, psoriasis or a fungal infection. The places in or on their body where these symptoms appear are significant. However, different parts of the body mean different things to different people. You cannot draw up a fixed list of symbolic illnesses and corresponding places on the body. Only the ill person could tell you what their illness means – and it does usually have a meaning. However, whatever the symptoms, they always point towards the problem of inner conflict. Resolve the inner conflict and the symptoms will disappear. The trickier the problem, the more severe the symptoms, but remember that the symptoms are there to allow you to bring your awareness to that spot.

Headaches

The biggest apparent cause of headaches is eating or drinking something that disagrees with the individual. Everyone knows how alcohol can cause a hangover and a headache but few know that drinking tea also results in headaches. Sometimes, for people who drink a lot of tea, even stopping drinking can cause a temporary headache. The solution is easy: stop the tea/coffee/alcohol. Anyone who cannot stop has deeper problems involving addictive habits. Headaches are important symptoms. Taking painkillers abuses the body and is a way of deliberately ignoring the information which the body is trying to give you in order to keep you on the right track. The cause must be identified for the problem to be solved. Painkillers will only ever relieve symptoms, not tackle causes.

The head is always a crucial position in any organization, and that includes your body. If there is pain here (even after the removal of tea, coffee and alcohol), finding out what the pain in the head represents *for the sick person* is important. A healer may have many theories about what the head represents, but they are only theories. What is important is what the *patient* thinks it represents. This is because the patient alone holds the key to their own healing. In a sense, no one else can do the healing for them. All the healer can do is to listen and try to understand, alongside the patient, what the problem is and to mirror it energetically until it resolves itself.

Every symptom has a meaning for the sick person. The location of the problem and its nature is significant. It is similar with dreams, where the only really useful interpretation is the one made by the dreamer him/herself. Every figure is significant and every detail has meaning for the dreamer. Any meaning that other people try to impose on the dream is largely irrelevant and may confuse understanding.

Back pain and other back problems

The back or spine can be thought of in at least two different ways. Firstly, it is the place behind you, the past. Unresolved problems from the past could become lodged in the back, causing the person pain which, in turn, focuses the attention (possibly only subconsciously) on the past, unresolved problem. Secondly, the back could represent the support which the individual feels they have. If there isn't much support, the back could feel weak. (Remember: it is not the feeling of weakness that causes the back pain but the stuck energetic problem which causes both the feeling of weakness and the weak back.) Or the back could represent something else altogether. The point is not so much which part the back represents but that, whatever it represents, this representation has been created by the patient and contains a conflict.

Each patient creates their own links between psychological states and physical parts, via the vitality. These links are created by their own experiences and their culture and are unique to each individual. Although they are not directly linked, they are indirectly connected via the life force. With inner conflict comes distortion in the life force, the physical result of which becomes apparent in whichever part of the body is most significant to the patient.

Eczema

Whilst distortions in the life force only show up in symptoms that are particular to the individual, there are some illnesses which seem to be entirely predictable in their manifestation. Indeed, it is these illnesses which lead to the generalizations about health which have caused so many misunderstandings.

A Theory

My wife and I have proven to ourselves that eczema is a truly preventable disease for the majority of people. In a large number of people, dairy products are the main cause of eczema. Why is this? The skin is an organ of elimination, designed to eliminate liquids. If it tries to eliminate solids, eczema will develop because the solids do not fit and the skin has to break down for the solids to escape – this happens naturally and through scratching. Dairy products appear to fool the skin most easily, making the skin think that they are liquids when, in fact, they are solids. This could be because our first food, human milk, may be eliminated easily through the skin while cow's milk is different (it's designed for calves, for a start) but the body may not be able to detect this difference. When dairy products are totally eliminated from the diet, the eczema usually disappears completely. If it doesn't, it is usually because the person is using goat's milk or soya milk as a substitute. These can also result in eczema.

For most people, pasteurized milk is generally much harder to tolerate than unpasteurized (again, following Pasteur's theories has not been helpful!), and milk protein causes more problems than milk fat. Lactose (milk sugar) only causes problems for a minority who are specifically 'lactose intolerant'. When someone has eczema, all dairy products (from any animal) should be eliminated initially (including dairy products taken by breast-feeding mothers if the baby suffers from eczema). The ingredients list on every packet of food needs to be read to ensure that some form of dairy has not been added (in the form of whey powder, caseins, skimmed milk powder, milk solids, etc.). This is not an absolute cure because nothing has changed in the body, although the skin will heal. There is much evidence that dairy products do more harm than good to a large number of people and provide the 'maintaining cause' of many symptoms. Indeed, in several experiments, pasteurized milk fed to calves has been shown to produce adverse effects.

Even though the elimination of dairy products from the diet might alleviate all the symptoms of eczema, this is still not true healing. This is because the diagnosis of 'eczema' is based on recognizing a pattern of symptoms rather than the true cause: disordered life force. Symptoms are easy to change with drugs, which can make it look as if the disease has disappeared, but this is not the case if the disordered life force is still there. In fact, it is easy to eliminate the symptoms of a disease without understanding its cause. Many people do, of course, equate removal of symptoms with cure, but this is limited thinking which only stores up trouble for the future.

Tinkering with symptoms is not the solution to any disease – in the same way that taking vitamins doesn't make up for a poor diet, building better sea defences doesn't change global warming, turning the volume down on the television doesn't improve an awful programme, having an affair doesn't solve a bad marriage, and so on. But we all indulge in some of these activities because we can fool ourselves into thinking that they do have a positive effect.

Unfortunately, this is also the basis on which western medicine operates. While there is no understanding of the life force or vitality, western medicine will only be tinkering with symptoms.

Vaccinations have caused some diseases to apparently disappear; at least, some of the classic symptoms are not as widespread as they once were. The vaccinations teach the body in advance how to deal with the viruses. The body does a good job. Unfortunately, the disease is not only the symptoms: it is also the disordered life force, and this is not addressed by the vaccination. So the distorted life force, the disease, stays in place but the classic symptoms are not there to indicate that anything is wrong. What will happen? Actually, several different things can happen: the disease can be eliminated by the vitality of the patient or it can stay in place and get worse so that other symptoms start to show. The body's production of symptoms (for example, in the traditional childhood diseases), is its way of working through the disease process to a satisfactory resolution. With vaccinations, what were once acute diseases may be replaced by long-term, or chronic, ones. For example, it is not uncommon for children who have had the MMR vaccine to suffer with repeated ear infections and glue ear, often for years on end. The connection between the vaccination and the resulting illness is not usually made by the G.P., but any homeopath could give examples of this kind of pattern from their practice.

The body is always trying to get better, but when distortions occur in the life force, work is needed to restore the flow and we can be lazy or simply unsure of how to proceed without help.

Multiple Sclerosis

Without reference to the life force, diseases are difficult to discuss because, regardless of their name, they all have a similar cause: distorted life force brought on by inner conflict. However, some diseases are much more clearly energetic (i.e. energy-based) in nature. A splinter, for example, has a clear physical aspect and talking to a patient with a splinter about life force distortions doesn't make much sense (unless they get four or five splinters a day). Diseases that have a solely energetic cause are very difficult for western medicine to understand and treat but for the life force healer they are relatively easy to deal with. Multiple Sclerosis is one such disease. Western medicine claims that it attacks randomly because, without an understanding of vitality, that is how it appears. Actually, nothing in life acts randomly, although things which we do not understand may seem to. I believe that everything has a cause.

Having worked with many people diagnosed with MS, I now feel that I understand the disease. It is an energetic disease and one which only a human being can have. All the people I have seen with a diagnosis of MS have not known how to deal effectively with their emotions. Instead of working through them completely, they store them away and put a block up to prevent them from feeling, usually because they believe their problems are too difficult to deal with. A fair amount of stubbornness is needed to perform this task. Only human beings can do this. As with everything in life, whenever you do anything for sufficient time it begins to feel natural, as if it requires no effort. Not dealing with your emotions can be like this. As other emotional difficulties come along, the same method of dealing with them is used. Slowly but surely, the energetic block gets bigger. Eventually, it becomes so big and strong that it starts to affect the physical and mental states of the person. The person may still not feel what is going on until the distorted life force begins to have a more tangible and eventually debilitating effect on the functioning of the physical body. One of the interesting things about MS, and possibly every disease, is that the person who has it often believes that they can heal themselves. The truth is that they can. What they have to do is become aware of their own life force and the blocks which they have created.

With MS patients, I can feel the energetic block within them. I can also teach other people to feel it and I can teach people how to remove it. Taken seriously, this could change the treatment of MS dramatically. Incidentally, I can cause an energetic block to exist temporarily in someone who doesn't have MS, giving them a feeling of what it is like to have the disease – the body fails to respond to commands to move. It is not the de-myelination of the nerve that causes this paralysis; that comes later, and results from not using the body properly. I believe that this is a vivid way of demonstrating how changes in the flow of energy directly affect the physical functioning of the body.

I believe that curing someone of MS involves showing them how to remove the energetic block and, in turn, how to avoid allowing it to re-grow. This is relatively easy to do. I suspect, although I do not yet know for sure, that certain other diseases which are similarly energy-based (such as Parkinson's Disease and Motor Neurone Disease), could also be treated using this technique.

HIV/AIDS

I believe that it is possible to help all nameable illnesses with the Boulderstone Technique and even help some that have no name. I often get asked the question, 'Does this mean that it can help people with HIV/AIDS or cancer or any other "incurable" disease?'. Obviously, these 'incurable' diseases represent some kind of extreme for people. Perhaps the sheer number of people who have died from them plays its part; also, most people have had the experience of knowing someone with one of these diseases. The belief that no cure can possibly exist unless the doctors are offering it seems virtually unshakeable amongst the general public.

When I have worked with people who are HIV positive, I can feel a very specific form of distorted life force. I always say that the virus is not responsible for any disease since there are many people who have the virus but do not go on to have the associated symptoms, and this is also true of HIV. However, this does not mean that the HIV drugs will not work. They may work on the level of the virus but, if they do not touch the distorted life force, they are clearly not providing a permanent cure.

Does it matter that the HIV drugs do not cure but do, for a limited period, remove the symptoms? This is one of the most important questions in this book. Let me make the question more general: *Does it matter if the vaccination / antibiotics / steroids or other drugs take away the symptoms of the disease but leave in place the distorted life force?*

The answer, of course, is yes, it does matter. This is because the blueprint for the body, feelings and thought processes of the individual is their *flow* of life force. If it becomes distorted then the body, feelings and thought processes will become distorted. If the expression of the distorted life force is denied and the distorted life force stays in place, it will slowly create a bigger problem. Luckily, the body often heals itself naturally over time, especially during sleep when some of the patient's will, used to keep the illness in place, is relaxed. All medicine that is not designed to address the distorted life force will generally make the patient worse and confuse the body's messages concerning how to cure.

The same can be said for the planet; in this instance, the result is much starker. If the symptoms of global warming are dealt with, does this take away the disease? As in the human body, the symptoms cannot be completely eradicated. Flood barriers can be erected, sea defences can be strengthened, people can be re-housed but in no way does that resolve the problem. Only when the conflict between our desire to dominate nature and our realization that we are part of nature is resolved will the symptoms disappear.

Miasmas

Diseases without a name; the source of many illnesses.

People in stressful jobs often get 'burnt out'; they lose their energy, direction and *raison d'etre*. (I believe that, coincidentally, this is also the state of the western world). Other symptoms could include: tiredness (where sleep doesn't relieve); general aches and pains; headaches; and sluggishness, perhaps with a desire for stimulants. Western medicine may diagnose this as Myalgic Encephalomyelitis (ME) or Epstein Barr or plain old Post-Viral Fatigue Syndrome, but the cause is energetic and, as such, an orthodox physician will not be able to deal with it effectively. If the patient went to a physician a few hundred years ago, they may well have been told that they were possessed by an evil spirit. (Indeed, in some parts of the world, the same thing may be said today.) If this were the case, the treatment would be to go and see someone skilled in the removal of spirits, usually a holy person or shaman. Nowadays, few people know how to deal with this situation, yet the symptoms still exist. Patients generally go to doctors who, on the whole, have a very hard time with this sort of illness. In many cases, one of the *anti* drugs is prescribed. Actually, it is interesting that each and every one of the *anti* drugs has been prescribed to different patients in my practice who share the same diagnosis of ME. None of them have really helped. These drugs are all anti-life force and cannot offer a cure.

I have seen this state described in fiction: 'Another pointless morning. She lay in bed, unwilling to wake, having no desire to trudge through another day. The sky was a smothering blanket of grey. The greyness seemed to seep into everything in the room, washing out any possibility of joy. Her eyes were heavy and tired, her head felt like cotton wool, only more painful. She dragged herself out of bed and down the stairs. Various children that she felt no connection to called out in greeting, but the prospect of responding to them was too exhausting. How long had she been like this? Was it since her brother's suicide? Her mother's death when she was young? When she was in the grey cloud, it was impossible to remember any good times or, indeed, to expect any in the future, the way it is impossible to feel the heat of summer on a cold winter's day. The pills from the doctor couldn't touch the darkness. It felt like nothing could.' (Katharine Ball)

The 'grey cloud' is referred to in pre-modern medicine as a *miasma*. This *miasma* is defined in the Shorter Oxford English Dictionary as 'poisonous germs floating in the atmosphere'. Miasmas are surprisingly common. I can feel them as a shadow that lies beneath the surface energy. They are insidious in their ability to attach themselves to people. These are the real germ – packets of disordered life force attached to people but easily caught in the process of social interaction.

They are created during a stressful time through overwork, the flu or a strong emotional experience. When I started working directly with the life force, I often used to catch these miasmas which made me feel very tired and irritable. Surprisingly, my wife used to recognize when this had happened to me more easily than I did. Eventually, I learnt how to look for them and remove them from myself; my mood would lift instantly and the tired feeling would disappear. I now use this as the main criterion for testing people to whom I teach the Boulderstone Technique – their ability to deal with miasmas is a crucial indicator of their readiness to practise on others. All the skills you need in order to heal someone are contained within the ability to discover and remove any miasma that comes your way. Could this miasma also be the basis for the fictional vampire; a creature that feeds on human blood, itself a metaphor for vitality?

The healing principle

Symptoms and illness are your body's exclusive healing messages.

As soon as you are able to define your disease as *distorted life force brought on by inner conflict,* your cure will be within your grasp. Life force flows through everything; only the blocks which you put up to it cause your symptoms. This may happen because you confuse remembered pain with active pain (see the discussion of *Pain* earlier in this chapter). When you train yourself to be sensitive to the blocks to life force in yourself and others, you can help people who do not have that sensitivity. If, for example, a patient has panic attacks, you will be able to feel the effort they are expending in avoiding the experience of the remembered pain. At this point, what does the healer do, or what would you do? Would you break down their block? The answer is strange: you do all that you can to help them keep the block in place. You match the effort they are expending in not feeling the pain. This seems counter-intuitive, but doing it upsets the balance that the patient has in keeping the illness in place. The inner conflict that has been kept stable up until this point, is no longer stable. The life force flowing through the patient wants to heal them but it has been prevented from doing so by the patient's resistance towards the experience of 'remembered pain'. Then, as the healer, you gently increase the resistance. What then happens is that the patient's life force responds in order to keep things balanced. Then you slowly release the artificial block and the life force has the ability to do its healing work now that the block has been removed. The healer actually makes the minimum of effort; the patient does most of the work. They don't even need to be conscious because the life force is always awake.

Strong emotions may be felt and released as the life force does its work. The physical body may twist and contort and thoughts will come and go. In this way, panic attacks, or whatever the problem, are permanently removed.

The question now arises, 'What conditions can the Boulderstone Technique *not* help?' The answer is that it can help all problems that result from a distorted life force caused by inner conflict. In short, it has the potential to resolve all illnesses (with the exception of certain inherited disorders) and, furthermore, is a useful tool to transform your consciousness even if you do not believe that you are ill. Where you will end up is anybody's guess.

There is more to life force healing than this, however. The principles that hold true here also hold true for any organization that is controlled by a human being. Organizations can develop a distorted life force, which can only come from inner conflict. When management are pulling in different directions an 'illness' will result. The solution is not to shore up the products of the problem but to resolve the conflict itself.

Part 4: Solutions

Actually, there is only one solution – to allow the life force to flow freely.

Your plan

You can use this section to improve your health as well as your level of happiness. Ultimately, the path of increasing health and happiness is also the path to enlightenment. If you are taking steps in this direction, you are also allowing for your spiritual development, whether you 'believe in' these things or not. However, just reading about solutions is not enough: active participation is essential. The first step is to devise your plan for enlightenment, then put it into action and continually work with and modify it. Without having the 'end' in mind, it is difficult to move in the right direction. Putting your life in other people's hands and expecting them to find solutions for you is something that a lot of people want but it will not get you where you want to go. By all means get advice from as many people as possible (and there are many people willing to give it!), but don't spend more time getting the advice than putting it into practice.

Some of the following exercises take you to a place beyond thought. Occasionally, this can be counter-productive because you forget what you were meant to be doing. The inability to remember what you were doing causes you to keep repeating actions until they are remembered. A simple way around this is to write down what you are attempting in a journal. So, the first thing you need to do is to get a notebook or journal, and use this to remind yourself of what you have been doing and where you want to go. This journal needs to be continually updated.

Exercise Get a journal

Decorate it with symbols and pictures that mean something to you – give it some magic.

Every time you write in your journal, start with the date. It may not be useful now but in years to come, when you look back at it, you will be amazed at how far you have travelled in such a short time. You may also find that some things do not seem to change at all. Recording your endeavours will give you clarity about your life and the direction in which it is going.

Exercise Defining your direction

After writing the date, you need to write down a list of things you want under the following headings: Work, Relationships, Family, Spiritual, Physical.

Notice how these headings are just another definition of you. You can make up other headings or leave some out – there is no definitive list. I have not written any guidelines for your wants; just be true to yourself. If you want a Ferrari more than anything else and you think it will make you happy, then go for it. Initially, wishes may start off a bit egocentric, but as time goes by, they usually become more far-reaching. Doing this simple exercise gives you a direction, without which you tend just to want more of everything you have. You will find that, as time goes by, your wish-list changes. Check it weekly. Some of the things you wish for may happen very quickly, and you may find that you get them and then lose motivation. For example, when people come to my meditation classes, they sometimes say that they want peace of mind. Very often, they get their peace of mind in the first few weeks, forget how important this was to them, do not remember why they came to the class in the first place and eventually stop coming. Since discovering this, I now get everyone to write down their wishes for the future.

Finding 'the force'

I believe that finding and maintaining 'the force' is the single most important thing you need to do in this life. Knowledge of it maintains health and happiness.

Exercise Getting to know 'the force'

For this exercise you need the help of another person, at least for the first time you try it, so that you can get some physical feedback.

Sit on a stable chair and have your partner gently but firmly push your arm so that you are aware of how much effort you need in order not to be pushed over. Resist their push. Remember the effort you need to make in order to stay upright. (When they start to go over, most people smile. This is because they are moving from one realm to another. See Discrete Living-realms.)

Have your partner read the following to you. Complete each section and nod to your partner when you are ready to move on.

1. *Find the sense that tells you where your feet are. Just know where they are. Nod when you have done this and want to move on. (Don't take longer than five seconds.)*
2. *Keep that sense of your feet in mind, but now also find the sense that tells you where your knees are.*
3. *Keep those two in mind and find the sense that tells you where your hips are.*
4. *Keep all of that in mind and know where the roof of your mouth is.*
5. *You do not need to push back now, just decide that you are not going to move.*

Get your partner to gently push you again while being aware of where your whole body is. Ask your partner to slowly increase the strength of the push. Do not use your muscles to resist.

Feel the power of the force. No effort is needed to equal the strength you used to stop being pushed over. Watch how easy it is to lose awareness of it. Try not to. Also notice that while you maintain awareness of 'the force' your thinking slows. You are moving into the present.

Now swap over and read the instructions to your partner.

Getting 'the force' is a way of bringing you right into the present and, at the same time, helping you to know who you are, physically. This is what gives you the physical ability to resist the push without effort. When you also know who you are emotionally and mentally, you gain an emotional and mental strength as well. For the time being, though, we are just working with the physical body. To some extent, the other parts automatically come along with the physical body anyway.

Keeping an awareness of 'the force' should be your only aim in life. If you can do this, you will not have inner conflict; anything that you subsequently do will inevitably be what is exactly and uniquely right for you. The question arises, what things take you away from 'the force'? Just as keeping 'the force' prevents inner conflict from developing, so it is precisely inner conflict that will cause you to lose it. Look at how you personally lose contact with it in your life. Unless you are a professional sportsman, or someone else who concentrates intensely on the body as part of their everyday activities, you will probably lose awareness of 'the force' very easily. But how does this happen for you? If you can discover what causes you to lose awareness, you can use this knowledge to train yourself in ways to maintain it. Then you will have discovered your real teacher.

When you consciously experience 'the force', your awareness goes beyond thoughts and feelings – this makes it difficult to talk about. The rational mind even desires to trivialize it because it cannot understand it entirely and therefore believes it to be irrational and that it shouldn't exist. Having 'the force' can feel like you are not doing anything, until you start using it. Being pushed is a trivial example but it demonstrates 'the force' reasonably well. When it is used in conjunction with other activities, it is transformative and healing. Having 'the force' all the time is a powerful experience. If you can keep it through any activity then that activity will be greatly enhanced. Indeed, people try to obtain 'the force' when they train in a repetitive activity – whether that be learning a new piece of music or perfecting a run up for the long jump. If the people performing these activities know how to use 'the force', their performance becomes much improved.

Having 'the force' actually entails being aware of two forces. The first is the one that appears to give you strength, while the second is the one that keeps everything fluid. They are both present in equal measure when you have 'the force'. The one that keeps everything fluid is your life force. The other is your resistance to that life force. In a sense, it is a death force, death being an opposite to life. That said, in any battle the life force will always win over the death force. The death force is ego-based while the life force is beyond that. This is why human beings will always be able to improve if they can let go of their ego. I call this death force the *I-force*.

You cannot maintain 'the force' and tell a lie or have any form of inner conflict. This is the basis of the Boulderstone Technique; it can also be used as an indicator of what is right for you. When you can maintain 'the force' throughout the day, you will be one hundred percent healthy, one hundred percent happy and spiritually enlightened.

Outlined below are some practical exercises that are designed to allow you to experience the life force. The exercises will also teach you how to remove the blocks which we put up against it. Some of the exercises are taken from secret teachings but all require you to have 'the force'.

Exercise 'The force' and a lie

*Get 'the force'. You may need to refer back to the exercise
Getting to know 'the force' and find the sense that tells
you where your feet etc. are. Try to keep 'the force' while
thinking of a lie or inner conflict. You should find it is
impossible.*

Exercise 'The force' gives integrity

*If you play a musical instrument, try playing it with 'the
force'. It may be harder to play than usual. It may even
sound the same to you. Invite someone else to listen and see
if they can tell the difference.*

Exercise Physical exercise

*Depending on your age, some form of daily physical exercise
is important for your health. This should include a stretching
session and an aerobic session, all done with 'the force'.
Whatever exercise you choose, it should not be difficult, hard
or painful. More pain: less gain. Exercise is only sustainable
if it makes a positive contribution to your life. I once read
that physical exercise prolongs your life but only by the
amount of time you spend doing it. If this is the case, you
had better enjoy your time exercising or you will just make
your life more miserable. Ten minutes' walking each day is
sufficient if you are grossly out of shape, but if you can
handle this without a problem, add another ten minutes.
Start adding in a little jogging time and keep going until you
can easily jog for twenty to thirty minutes. As always, the
trick is not to progress too quickly. Acknowledge your
limitations and slowly push them back. The only thing that
will make you give up is the fact that you are expending too
much effort. But how much should you do? Luckily, you have
a built-in evaluation device. If you stay with 'the force' you*

know when you have done enough. Very often, it will tell you to stop and, when it does, you should listen. When you don't listen to 'the force', calamity will surely follow.

No pain: only gain

It is important to your health to have a daily practice of some description, but it is equally important that this daily practice requires as little effort as possible. This is because making an effort is not sustainable. Effort is needed to overcome inertia but, generally, daily practice should be effort-free. If you look at the things in your life that you already do on a daily basis, you will see that they do not require much effort. For example, a daily activity of mine, as for most people, is brushing my teeth. Nowadays, it happens without my appearing to make any effort: I just know it has to be done and I do it. What surprises me is that for many years I valued my teeth more than my mind. By that I mean that a daily mind-cleanse is just as important for your health as is cleaning your teeth. Another daily activity of mine is going for a run, and, surprisingly, although I sweat this activity also requires very little effort. When you have 'the force' constantly, every thing you do is without effort.

Your daily practice needs to include exercise on a mental/emotional/spiritual level as well as on a physical level. If it does not, the baggage of your life will begin to build up and before long you will be lost in a mess of your own inertia. You do not need to spend a lot of time on the exercise but you do need to spend *some* if you are to stay healthy.

Food choices and 'the force'

Getting healthy requires that you know how food affects you, especially since your appetite for food is governed more by your ego than by your physical needs. As a race, it has taken us millions of years for our bodies to develop and modify to such a degree that we are now able to eat virtually anything. In contrast, it has taken the multibillion-dollar food industry and our own greed just a few years to turn packaged food into something which, although our bodies find useless, our egos feel is essential. Processed food, eaten exclusively, causes problems for most people. Unprocessed food generally does not.

A lot of the 'facts' which we have about food have been discovered by people who are not aware of life force. For example, it is commonly believed that no one can survive for more than three days without water. And yet, *breatharians* go through a process whereby they do not drink for seven days and do not eat for a lot longer still. These *breatharians* have been thoroughly checked out and seem to be genuine. They do not eat (or eat very little) sometimes for years at a time. This does not fit with current scientific thinking, which makes it difficult to believe, but waiting until science catches up with reality seems like burying your head in the sand.

While I cannot claim to have practical experience of not eating for months at a time, I do know some things about food. For example, fasting for short periods makes me feel better, stronger and more alive. Also, when people are ill they often stop eating and I believe this helps them to get better more quickly. A lot of the food we eat has a more negative than positive effect on the body – making us tired, sluggish, constipated or loose, bloated, uncomfortable and lacking in energy. This may be due to one of several factors: food intolerances, unhealthy or highly-processed food, or simply bad eating habits.

Through my healing work, I have become more sensitive to everything around me, especially my life force. I can turn off this sensitivity but I prefer not to. I use it to help me. For example, before I eat something new I get 'the force' and then place my finger on the food and monitor how that feeling changes. I can detect precisely how my body is reacting to any food and know there and then what is good for me and what is not. Of course, I have the human reaction of denial built in and so it has taken me a long time to reach a point where I am prepared to admit that drinking alcohol and eating chocolate both cause me problems. Everyone is different and you may be fine with these substances. However, through this process I discovered that I have a problem with vanilla which causes me to get mouth ulcers. I do not believe that I could have found this out by any other method. Nowadays, I do not need to look on the label to know whether a food is good for me or not: I can just hold the packet and feel its effects.

This sensitivity, which we all have and can all develop further, is the basis of a therapy called kinesiology. A kinesiologist tests the strength of muscles (or, more accurately, the life force flowing through the muscles) when the body comes into contact with different substances, usually foods. Muscle weakness suggests that there is an intolerance. Western medicine can only detect true allergies which manifest when actual, measurable antibodies have been formed. Since intolerances (as opposed to full-blown allergies) cannot be measured in a laboratory, they are mostly dismissed as insignificant by the medical profession. This is despite the fact that they are often the major cause (or, at least, a highly significant causal factor) in the case of eczema, irritable bowel syndrome, rhinitis, sinusitis, colitis, bloating, acne, mouth ulcers, glue ear, hay-fever, asthma and a whole host of other 'clogging' illnesses.

The test which the kinesiologist makes is not one that can be made by a machine. It is better than that. It is not totally objective – the state of the tester has, for a long time, been known to be significant. If the kinesiologist is clear in their thinking then they will get a clear answer. If they are confused or prejudiced then they will get a confused or prejudiced answer. This can also be used to advantage by a very 'clear' tester who can introduce his or her own ideas and see how the results change. For example, the tester can ask the life force, 'Can this be changed?' or 'Will this intervention help?'. Without conscious participation or speech the patient 'knows' the answer and the muscle will respond appropriately. What a shame it is that this method of testing is disregarded by Western medicine, basically because it cannot be performed by a machine.

People get used to feeling weakened by certain foods and drinks, such as tea, coffee and alcohol. In muscle testing, these drugs nearly always switch a person off. By that I mean that their muscles become weak. People often associate this feeling with relaxation and welcome it, but really these substances are poisons to the life force and to the body.

Food problems often figure highly for patients with long-term chronic illness, not least because their vitality has taken such a battering that the patient cannot hear it when their life force says, 'Do not eat that.' This is one way in which a Boulderstone Technique practitioner can be helpful. However, if you use your life force to direct you in what to eat and how to live, you will never be let down.

Exercise Food sensitivity

Put aside five different sorts of food – such as sugar, wheat, cow's milk or cheese, alcohol, coffee and perhaps some other substances which you are not sure are good for you or not. (It does not matter what the substances are wrapped in as 'the force' works through glass, plastic and paper.) In addition, get hold of some red food colouring or artificial sweetener. Lie or sit in a comfortable place and relax for a few moments and get 'the force'. Have the food substances within easy reach and pick up each one in turn. Feel the effect each one has on you. Each will be different in some way. Some you may not be able to detect clearly, some may make you feel relaxed, some strong and some weak. Your body knows which are good for you and which are not.

Next, try some fruit and vegetables. Do not pre-judge the results. You may be pleasantly surprised by your ability to feel differences in your responses to these different substances. Some people can act on the strength of the results they find. Others have to go to see a 'professional' and pay money before they believe the results.

If you do change your diet, keep testing yourself because the results will not stay fixed forever. Make sure that you take responsibility for whatever you put in your mouth. Do not pass that responsibility on to your doctor, healer, mother, father, partner or child.

Methods of resolving inner conflict

Regardless of the method, you must start from where you are. It doesn't matter if you are going to change your diet, do some exercise or start meditating – you must start from where you are now and not from where you would like to be.

Everyone who has an ego, has a built-in realm (see *The Realms as the Basis for Inner Conflict*) or structure and therefore a potential for inner conflict. But it is still possible to stay healthy if you know how to move beyond and through your realms. To break habits of a lifetime, you need to know how to use the two contradictory forces I described earlier. The first force is the ability to hold on to something – I call it the Will, which relates to the *I-force* – while the second is the ability to let go of something – which I call Love (or sometimes Non-attachment) and relates to the life force.

The instant that we get lost in a realm is the instant that our world comes into existence; this occurs when we let the I-force dominate. Inner conflict is the cause.

Simply destroying the realm is not the solution because the realm that decided to do the destroying will take on the problems and karma of the realm which it destroys. For example, giving up an addiction cannot be achieved just by removing the addictive substance. Although giving it up will certainly bring to the surface the underlying reasons for the addiction, if these are not dealt with then the patient is still effectively addicted. The only solution is to find the realm's inner conflict. You will find and work through the realm's inner conflict only if you know how to get and maintain 'the force' (see *Finding 'the force'*). One way to uncover and deal with inner conflict is through yoga.

Yoga

Two thousand years ago, Patanjali wrote: *Yoga is the science of resolution of inner conflict* (my translation). He then went on to explain all the steps you need to take in order to resolve that inner conflict.

Yoga is an amazing exercise but one that is often misunderstood. Certainly, there are many different kinds of yoga but, in their different ways, they are all essentially aiming to do the same thing: resolve inner conflict. However, some of them have lost their way over time and have become distorted to the point of now being almost exclusively physical.

Yoga has not always involved physical exercise. It originated as a spiritual exercise, used to connect oneself to God, which is another way of saying connecting 'heaven' and 'earth'. Nowadays, yoga has become more of a stretching exercise with only the gentlest of nods to its past. However, yoga is really much more than this.

Yoga, at its best, is not about getting into perfect physical poses, but about asking you questions of an energetic nature which you have to answer. Some of this is done via the physical body. All bodies have a physical limit – no one is infinitely flexible. When you are moving into a yoga pose, you will reach the end of comfortable movement. Yoga then asks you the question, 'What do you do now?' You answer in one of several ways. You may try to go deeper into the pose and ignore the pain; you may try to escape by coming out of the pose; or you may just stay where you are and hold the pose. Whatever you do, and the way that you do it, is the real practice of yoga. So the stiffer your joints are, the better off you are since you will have more to work with. In fact, you could feel sorry for the trained dancers who are so flexible that they can lie down easily along their outstretched legs, for they are much less likely to understand what I am talking about.

We tend to make associations between our feet (or base chakra) and the earth, and also between the top of our head and 'heaven'. This may be simply because we walk upright but, whatever the reason, yoga exploits this association so that when we can be aware of the connection between our feet (or base chakra) and the top of our head, we may also be aware of the connection between 'heaven' and 'earth'. Yoga poses are designed to facilitate this connection.

Most men tend to give up yoga because they have a tendency to want to just push through all the pain barriers to be the best in the class. When this approach is taken, whether by men or women, injuries very often follow and thus the person will be forced to stop. This is a form of self-inflicted violence which needs to be looked at separately. Women tend not to have such a competitive streak and generally stay with yoga for longer, learning either directly or indirectly the subtleties of the exercise.

When you are physically pushed to your limit in yoga, wherever that limit may be, there is a tendency to focus automatically on the flow of life force; if you listen to its guidance, you will not push yourself too far. (You will know when you have gone too far as you will hurt yourself). This is one reason why you may stop breathing in a pose – it helps you to listen. The exhortation by yoga teachers to 'keep breathing' overrides what our bodies are saying to us. I believe that it is better to ignore this advice – you will not die – and follow the subtle movement of energy. The life force is more in evidence at these edges and is experienced as the fluid state described above. In yoga, you have the opportunity to examine the possibilities of how you act and react in difficult positions. Because you are working with your life force, you are also automatically practising mentally and emotionally, so that when you are pushed to your limit 'in the real world', be it physically or mentally, you already have some experience to draw upon and can act with more awareness. Some say that this is a nice side-effect but I believe it to be the main reason yoga came into existence. Actually, you don't even need to be aware that this is what you are doing, which is another reason why yoga is such a marvellous exercise.

So, one of the main points of yoga is to bring to your attention your physical, and therefore energetic, restrictions so that you can deal with them. You need 'the force' with you when you practise yoga so that you can keep the life force/I-force balance. If you maintain 'the force' while practising then you will get mental, emotional and spiritual benefits as well, since the life force underlies everything. But you have a choice: if you wish, you can go back to bed.

The secret postures and exercises of yoga

Most people appear to enjoy being privy to information that is denied to others, probably because it gives them a feeling of power. However, the secrets in this book are not those kind of secrets. The secrets described here are actually more profound than that. 'Secret' here means 'difficult to remember'. When you are in pain and yet manage to find a way out of the pain, you would think that you would remember how you did it but, in reality, it is very easy to forget. Forgetting happens because true health, and happiness, happens beyond thoughts and feelings and, in that space when healing has happened, there is no memory of it either. Memory requires thoughts and feelings. The secret healing techniques take you to a place beyond inner conflict and, in so doing, to a place beyond memory.

There are certain postures and other yogic activities that are excellent at dealing with inner conflict. Of course, they are the ones that seem to produce the most inner conflict themselves. Your job as a yoga practitioner is to maintain 'the force' throughout the whole of the exercise and through doing this to learn how to maintain 'the force' and awareness all the time.

Salute to the Sun

The first exercise is the 'Salute to the Sun'. Most yoga practitioners I have spoken to believe that it is an exercise which should be performed at sunrise. Indeed, that is a good time to perform it, except that the exercise is more concerned with your internal sun or Self (see *Understanding Death* for description of Self) rather than the external sun. The 'Salute to the Sun' is a series of exercises that basically bend the back backwards and forwards a number of times. If you can maintain 'the force' while performing this exercise then you will have taken 'the force' to the next level. Knowing where you are physically in the world gives you physical strength. Knowing where you are emotionally and mentally makes you strong in those areas also. The 'Salute to the Sun' exercise stimulates you both mentally and emotionally. Try a simplified version of it now: just arch your back and stretch into that arch. You can store the day's problems in your spine; arching backward and maintaining 'the force' begins to clear them out. Most people know this quite instinctively.

Exercise Salute to the Sun/Self

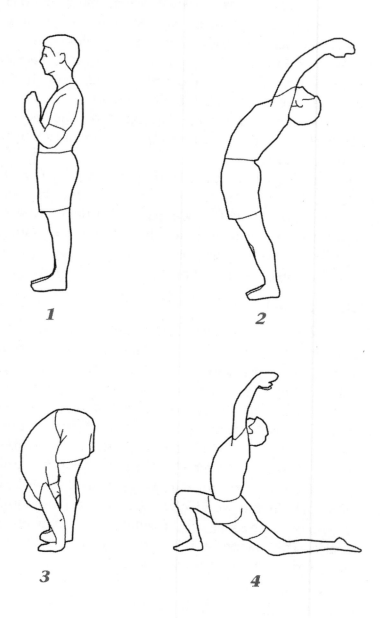

1   2

3   4

Salute to the Sun, continued

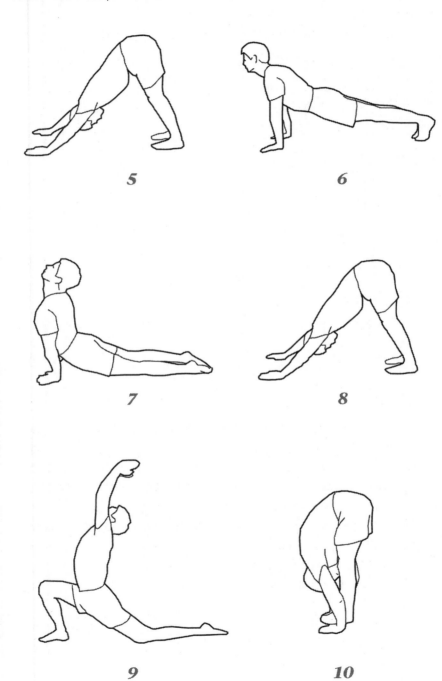

5

6

7

8

9

10

Salute to the Sun, continued

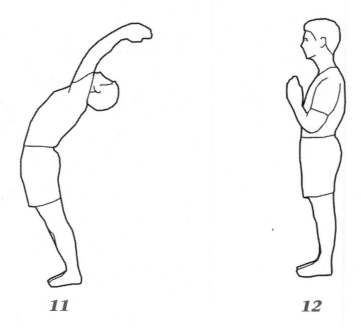

11   12

Maha Mudra

The next exercise also focuses on the back, and is called *Maha Mudra* (translated as '*The Great Attitude/Posture*'). It is described in the yogic text *Hatha Yoga Pradipika* (which just means 'Explanation of Yoga') as being able to destroy all illness, old age and death. Now, that is quite a claim for a single posture! Clearly, on the surface, the claim cannot be true. However, this text was written by people concerned with the truth so it should not be dismissed before attempting to understand that to which they were alluding. In order to do this, you need to get into the posture.

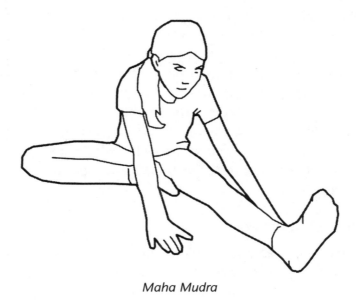

Maha Mudra

Exercise **Maha Mudra**

Place the heel of the left foot into the perineum and straighten the right leg in front of you. Personally, I have found that it does not make much difference whether the left knee is pointing upwards or to the side – both are technically Maha Mudra. *All yoga postures are difficult to some degree – that is the point of them – but if you need to sit on a cushion, that is totally acceptable. You now stretch forward and take hold of the right foot, or as near to it as you can. You need to look for the physical resistance; the sooner you get it, the better. Now concentrate on getting 'the force' and, as your head and neck and spine begin to get stretched, you will notice that wherever you store your difficulties is brought into your awareness to be dealt with. Maintaining 'the force', without force, brings you right into the moment and 'destroys illness, old age and death'. This is called 'raising Kundalini' by some.*

Keeping the spine 'clear' brings you directly into the present; in the present there is no inner conflict and therefore no disease, old age or death. This points to a state of being which has been described before. Living in the realm of the present, and only in the present, means that there is no conscious thought of disease, old age or death. Only the ego gets upset at this point and starts saying things like, 'What about my pension?' or, 'I won't get anything done in that state.' If you can get to the point where there is no inner conflict, everything that needs to be done will get done, including your pension.

Kapalbhati Pranayama

Pranayama means energy development (prana meaning life force) that very often involves using the breath and breathing. The next yogic exercise looks like a straightforward breathing exercise and, although it is often treated as such, in reality, as with most yoga exercises, it is designed to clear inner conflict. (Kapalbhati is Sanskrit and can mean 'clear head perception'.) When you breath out vigorously through your nose while maintaining 'the force', the focus for your attention moves to anywhere between the rear of your nose and the top of your head. When awareness is cloudy between these two areas then clarity of 'heaven' is impossible.

Exercise Kapalbhati Pranayama

> First, find a stable sitting posture. This can be in a chair, if necessary. Place your hands on your knees or thighs – whichever is more comfortable – and now find 'the force'. If you do not find 'the force', you may still be doing the exercise but it will have absolutely no value. Now breathe in and out through the nose, forcing the out-breath (nearly snorting it out) by contracting the abdomen. The in-breath should be allowed to happen naturally. Breathe at about the rate of one cycle per second. Your aim is to maintain 'the force' throughout – bear in mind that the exercise is

designed to cause you to lose 'the force'. In solving the problems of maintaining 'the force', you learn the inner meaning of Kapalbhati.

Never force any yoga exercise; keep going until you are aware that you have lost 'the force'.

Contrary to what many books say, *pranayama* does not build up life force in your system. What it does is remove the blocks (brought about by inner conflict) which you have created so that it appears that you have more life force. The point is that you are already enlightened under your clothes (as the Bible might say) and it is only your inner conflict that gives you the impression that you are energy-poor.

The exercise above is designed to clear the blocks that get stuck in the head area. It is impossible to say what sort of blocks these may be because they are different for everyone. Personally, I store over-exertion, which is violence towards myself, in my neck area. I store conflict from not doing the 'right' thing at the back of my head on a level with my eyes. Both of these areas get stimulated through *Kapalbhati* and then I resolve them through focused awareness (see *Removing a Block*).

Ujjayi Pranayama

The throat area is another place that gets used for storage of unresolved inner conflict. *Kapalbhati* is not that efficient at focusing on this area; another *pranayama* can be used instead. *Ujjayi* means 'victorious' and is described below. The exercise itself has a built-in conflict which can mirror a person's energetic conflict. This is the same principle that is expressed in the homeopathic phrase 'like cures like'.

Exercise Ujjayi Pranayama

Breathe in and out through your nose. At the same time, restrict your throat slightly so that you sound like a heavy breather from a horror movie. As before, the idea is to stimulate a problem which then has to be dealt with. By maintaining the breath, you automatically maintain awareness and allow yourself to process conflict.

This exercise can be performed on its own or in combination with a yogic pose or even while meditating.

There is no set number of times you should practise this exercise, or any other exercise. You are not trying to become the world's best at heavy breathing. The idea is to clear away your inner conflicts – firstly, by stimulating them and then maintaining the force.

Abdominal breathing

You can use abdominal breathing in the same way as *Kapalbhati* and *Ujjayi* to show you the conflicts that you have stored lower down in the spine. This area, from the bottom of your rib cage to your perineum, is usually a place in which people store their 'earthy' problems. Physically, these might show up as sexual dysfunction, piles, bladder problems, conception problems, digestive disturbances, and so on. The solution is always the same: reveal the problem by doing abdominal breathing, feel the energetic disturbance, discover the inner conflict that is holding it in place and then use 'the force' to dissolve it. This is the solution to all of life's problems!

Pranayama techniques can be enhanced by retaining the breath at different stages. Retaining the breath after inhaling increases the holding on (I-force) aspect while retaining the breath after exhaling increases the letting go (life force) aspect. Your own experiments will always bear fruit.

We tend to hold our conflicts energetically along our spine. However, they are not located in the physical spine, for if they were, we could cut them out with surgery. Actually, they are not held in the physical body at all (another reason why science cannot handle the concepts) but we do have access to them through the body using an inner sense. Problems will occur if we believe that this inner sense is a physical reality.

Mudras

Mudras are yogic poses for the hands. They are designed to stimulate different feelings in you. Your job is to keep 'the force' while you allow the feelings to come and go so that any feelings that have not been completely dealt with from past problems can be activated. Keeping 'the force' allows you to process the problems.

Exercise Mudras

> In a comfortable seated position, get 'the force' and become aware of how you feel. Next, touch together your forefinger and thumb of each hand and notice how your feelings change. Initially, hold the pose for between five and ten seconds. Maintain 'the force' and move the thumb to the second finger of each hand. You should be able to feel a difference in where you are focusing and a corresponding shift in your feelings and thoughts. Keeping 'the force' while bringing up suppressed feelings is the point of the exercise. Continue through all the fingers of both hands.
>
> Write up what you have felt in your journal. If you do not feel anything, just accept that mudras are not for you at the moment.

There are many different mudras and each can change the way you are feeling. It is then up to you to keep 'the force' while those changes occur. The purpose of mudras is not just to change your mood. Try these one at a time.

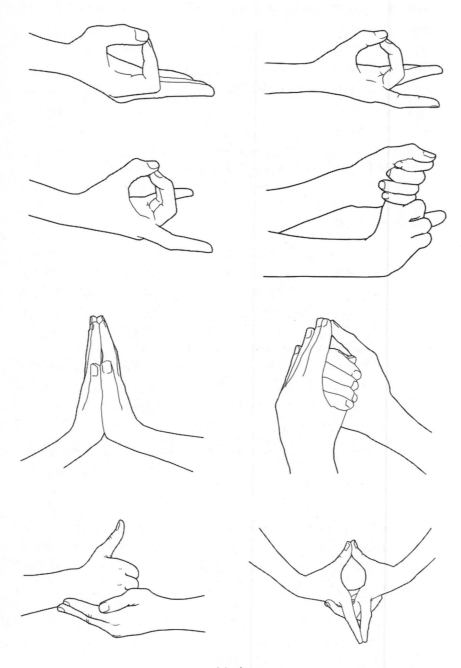

Mudras

Most yoga practitioners have come across *mudras* but very few use them on a regular basis. It would appear that they are generally not considered to be powerful. But they are as powerful as you want them to be. *Mudras* are often used by hypnotherapists as a way of releasing a previously stored state so that, when you take up a particular hand-shape, you change the way you feel. A yoga practitioner uses the associations you already have with your fingers while a hypnotherapist will create new ones. Neither is more effective than the other but the hypnotherapist is more conscious of what they are doing. If you accept the associations that you have already made with your fingers, you will be able to heal all your problems using different *mudras*.

Exercise Thoughts, feelings and your heart

This exercise is designed to show you that mudras (and therefore all yoga postures) are as powerful as you want them to be.

Find a comfortable seated posture, on the floor or in a chair. Get 'the force' and keep it. Notice how you are feeling and put your hands together in a prayer position in front of your heart. Notice what comes up for you. Now place your hands on your thighs, still maintaining 'the force'.

Now become aware of your thoughts, all of your thoughts, thoughts about what you are doing. Do not judge the thoughts, just be aware of them. Now, as well as you can, move all the thoughts into your right hand resting on your right thigh. Next, you need to become aware of your feelings. Give yourself as long as you need but do not get distracted. Place your feelings into your left hand. Now, start to bring your hands together in the same prayer position as before but this time realize that your thoughts and feelings are coming together in front of your heart. Bring your hands together slowly over a period of ten seconds or more.

Notice how different the exercise is from before.

The same is true for reflexology, a therapy designed to heal the whole person through working on the feet. According to reflexologists, different areas of the foot represent different parts of the person. Working on the feet through touch stimulates the corresponding part on the whole person. But how are the correspondences created? They are not fixed, for different schools of reflexology use different correspondences. As always, it is the patient that creates the structure (although people from the same culture will have similar correspondences). The best therapists are aware of this fact. Academic, or scientific learning, is not the key to being a good therapist, even if all the professional registering bodies believe that it is. The best therapist will have something that is immeasurable – awareness of their life force. They do not need to know anything else, for the flow of life force is all a person is.

Mantras and affirmations

A mantra is a phrase that is repeated over and over again while trying to maintain 'the force'. Mantras are usually written in Sanskrit. Sanskrit is a magical language because with it you can express ideas that are just not available in other languages. But what would happen if the mantra was written in English or your native language? Would it lose its power? My belief is that all spiritual exercises are only effective if they produce a difficulty for the practitioner to overcome. If you do not know what you are chanting, because it is in a language that is foreign to you, all that is left is the rhythm of the phrase. Rhythmic phrases can have an hypnotic effect on people – and maintaining 'the force' in this mental state is obviously useful – but understanding the words could easily be more powerful.

Affirmations are the western magical tradition's version of mantras. Affirmations are used in two distinct and different ways. The first is to find a sentence that is not true about yourself but which you would like to be. You then keep repeating it until it becomes true. An affirmation that is commonly used is, 'I am getting better and better in every way.' Unfortunately, this *can* work but only if you never stop saying it; you have to pound it into yourself. This is the violent method.

There is another way to use affirmations which is more effective, much less violent and much more in tune with working with the life force. You still find a sentence about yourself which you do not believe to be true but which you would like to be. However, as you say the sentence, it focuses your awareness on all the reasons why you believe it isn't true. You then deal with them by staying aware of the resulting inner conflict. In fact, you heal the disbelief that you are not what you wish for. When you can say the affirmation and maintain 'the force', the whole universe will be behind you.

When you construct your affirmation, it is important that it does not contain a negative. This is because the realm where your affirmation becomes true for you is beyond duality. Negatives lose their meaning when there is no duality. For example, if your affirmation is 'I do not want to be fat,' the realm where this is true actually hears, 'I want to be fat.' This is probably not what you intend! The way to resolve this problem is to be grateful for what you want; your affirmation might be, 'I am grateful for being slim.' You then deal with the inner conflict which may result. When you maintain 'the force' while repeating your affirmation, you will find that it is true.

Mantras take this one step further by dealing with spiritual matters rather than mundane ones. They do not need to be expressed in an unfamiliar language but, when they are, the effect is enhanced because it allows you to create a more complete picture in your imagination than you do when relying on words that you know. No mantra has any intrinsic power beyond that which you give it: however, each one uses basic sounds that often carry a profound meaning, whether or not you are conscious of it.

A favourite mantra is the *Gayatri Mantra* which is said to have been chanted continuously, without a break, for hundreds of years. In just a few syllables, this mantra contains a method of understanding yourself completely, as long as you maintain 'the force' while chanting.

Exercise Gayatri Mantra

> *Om bhûr, om bhuvaha, om swaha, om maha, om janaha, om tapaha, om satyam,*
>
> *om tat savitur varenyam*
>
> *bhargo devas ya dhîmahi*
>
> *dhiyo yo nah prachodayât*
>
> *The first half refers to the seven chakras or realms which constitute a complete person. The second half praises the creator of the universe and then goes on to say that the creator is within us.*

You need to experience the power of mantras yourself, by using them. Their power comes from resolving your inner conflict and setting free the creative power of the universe.

Miracles and magic

As a human being you are powerful. You can change the world with your thought. Indeed, mantras and affirmations change the world, and miracles and magic are just an extension of that. This is also why people pray – when they ask God for something, they are making it more important. In fact, answers to prayer (miracles, in other words) happen regularly. You may have experienced one or many yourself; in fact, I would be surprised if you haven't. They come from the least expected quarter and they come about because you ardently desire something and the universe obliges.

When consciousness changes, the effects of that change are felt in the physical world. In order to get what you want, you have to change your consciousness in the right way. There are many ways, but I will explain here one of the simplest methods that has worked for me.

In order to manifest anything, you must first get and maintain 'the force'. This gets you focused. Just wishing for something is not powerful enough. If you thank the universe for the thing that you want, even though you do not yet have it, you bypass a host of problems. Then you must go about your daily business without creating a break in consciousness. And that is it. Children do it naturally, especially at Christmas and their birthdays. If there is no break in consciousness, whatever you want will manifest.

This is the basis of the magic performed by witches and wizards. There is nothing evil about it; I am sure everyone has wished for something at least once in their life. However, there is a problem with doing it.

The problem with magic and consciously-directed miracles is that they also change the person performing them. The person 'creating' the miracle believes that the thing which they have created is important or valuable to them, when the truth of it is that its essential nature is emptiness. It is only by giving your 'self-created' riches away that you can 'enter the kingdom of heaven'. Some rich people understand this and will be happy. Some rich people do not understand this and are unhappy. What you eventually have to understand is that whatever you think you own is in fact theft and an encumbrance. By giving your possessions away, in your head at least, you free yourself up. Personally, I perform a daily rite where I 'put' all the things I think I possess into a stick of incense which I light, offering it to the universe. I 'put' into the incense everything I think I own as well as things which I know I don't really own but might think I do, such as my children and even my relationships (just calling them 'my' makes it clear that I think I own them). This act, which is performed afresh each day and doesn't become a meaningless ritual, frees up my ability to 'pass through the eye of a needle'. Creating anything makes you the god of the realm in which it exists. If you do not offer it to the universe, there is a danger that you will become stuck in this realm. When the rich man believes that he has created his wealth he will be stuck in that realm, unable to get to heaven.

Magic creates but comes with a price. As you learn how to meditate, so you are 'offered' psychic riches which take you away from your true goal. It is very easy for your ego to accept the prizes but then you will be side-tracked, losing your direction. It is better to meditate for its own sake – can you do that?

Meditation – The way to total happiness

Meditation is another branch of yoga. It is the best way to get to know yourself. For this very reason, it is probably the hardest. I meet many people who say that they cannot meditate because their thoughts will not stop, but this is the whole point. At the beginning of the yoga section, I said that yoga brings up your difficulties in order for you to deal with them; the same is true for meditation. It will bring up problems for you to solve. If your standard method of dealing with problems is to run away then you will learn very little and carry on with your life as it is. You have a choice. If you sit and watch your thoughts, you may see that they slow down.

The best and most basic meditation involves simply acquiring and maintaining 'the force'. That is all that is needed. It can be done at any time, any place and for any length of time, the length of time being dependent on what you are trying to achieve. Only a shift of realm will take you away from 'the force'. However, sometimes, just sitting down without knowing what you are doing can seem a little daunting; splitting up the procedure into smaller, more manageable pieces makes it easier. This is why there are many different methods of meditation and indeed different spiritual practices. These smaller, more manageable pieces require the creation of realms, the very things which you need to try to overcome, but if you are aware of this fact and keep them to a minimum then you can use them to your advantage. Whatever method or realm you use to gain partial enlightenment, that method or realm will eventually have to be dropped – for enlightenment is without boundaries.

The way to total happiness and health is easy: all you have to do is start from where you are and find the path through all your realms which does not end in a break in consciousness (see *Breaks in Consciousness*). To do this, you need to know when to hold on and when to let go, or how to employ Love and Will or, to put it yet another way, how to use life force and I-force -this is the same as maintaining 'the force' throughout the realms.

There is no one, external structure which can be applied to a human being as the basis for a therapy or path to enlightenment (and happiness) that will always work for everyone. Or, as Krishnamurti put it, 'There is no method to un-condition you.'

There are many ways to total happiness but, in the end, you have to find your own way by yourself. If you learn from another person how to be, you must totally assimilate what they have told you so that you can 'forget' it. It is only through 'forgetting' that you can learn it properly, otherwise you will just be a follower of rules. As a therapist, what I do is show the patient the structure which they have set up and which is causing them to be ill. The patient makes the decisions and their life force does the rest.

Although I have made the point that structures can cause problems, there is a common link between most structured religions and life force therapies. As I have mentioned before, we move our consciousness through realms, which are self-created. However, two of these realms are at the extremes of our consciousness and common to most spiritual traditions, even though they may go by different names in each.

The first is the 'earth' or the material realm. This is where everything that is physical exists. This is what comes into existence after creation and is the realm of the scientist. The other extreme realm is the realm of 'heaven'. The purpose of all spiritual traditions is to show you how these realms may be joined so that you can move your consciousness from one to the other without a break; to bring heaven to earth. This is their only purpose. When you can do this you will have total health and total happiness. Some religions teach that you can only reach heaven after you are dead – even if that is true (and since nobody knows with any certainty what happens after death), you could take that to mean 'death of the ego', in which case you can at least practise while still alive. (Incidentally, suicide falls into the category of destroying a realm.)

Whenever there is a description of how the world came into existence, in reality it is an attempt to show you how to move from one realm to another. There are many of these stories in the Bible. In Genesis, it happens in seven days. In the Gospel according to John (see free translation in *Discrete Living-realms*), it happens with a single word. Some believe in a big bang, whilst others believe that the universe is the dream of a god. The methods different traditions provide for making this connection are culturally dependent and so many stories come into existence, each one helping with an aspect of this journey.

When 'heaven' and 'earth' are connected within you, you understand how the physical world (including your own body) comes into existence, in this moment, and you are at one with 'the force'. This is the basis of total happiness and, as I see it, the sole purpose of all religions and all therapies including western medicine. It is what everyone has been after since the beginning of time.

We all already have the connection within us; if we believe we are not enlightened, it is only because we have put up blocks and created prejudices that cloud that knowledge. But to sit down and remove those blocks can appear to be a difficult process. And so we make it easier by splitting up the distance between 'heaven' and 'earth'. We create a structure which allows us to take the necessary baby steps that get us there in the end.

The number of staging-posts you create between 'heaven' and 'earth' is up to you. You don't need to set up any unless you find it difficult. But then who doesn't find it difficult at times?

One of the most obvious staging-posts lies at the mid-point between 'heaven' and 'earth' and is called many things by different traditions and therapies. Some of its names include: the Self, the Higher Self, the Christ Centre, the Buddha, the Heart Centre. It is a place beyond thoughts, beyond feelings and beyond the body. It is a place of 'emptiness'. Why emptiness? Because you have left behind thoughts and feelings so there is nothing to tell you about this place. And yet it exists.

It is essential that this place becomes familiar for all those wanting happiness. This is the place to which Jesus Christ was referring when he said, 'You have to pass through me to get to the kingdom of heaven.' Because it is a place of 'emptiness', you can take no thoughts or feelings there. This is a drawback for some people as they start to panic when their thoughts go silent; they think that they are going mad. Fear of this place is where panic attacks and schizophrenia can come from. Another reason that some people will not allow themselves into this 'emptiness' is a feeling of guilt which they cannot relinquish. Feelings of guilt lie at the heart of anyone who thinks that they have done wrong. However, these feelings have been put in place by that person alone.

When you can let go of all your thoughts, feelings and judgements, you will be able to move to this 'emptiness', this Self, halfway between 'heaven' and 'earth', a place of rest. But if you cannot let go of your thoughts then you may need to set up another staging-post between 'earth' and Self. In some traditions, these staging posts have been called *chakras*. They are created by the individual who uses them but they have no objective existence. You may assign colours and other attributes to them if you wish, but it is unnecessary and will ultimately only slow your progress. This is because they have more relevance in the traditions from which they come – here in the west, we do not have the same kind of master/disciple relationship and less need to communicate the ideas in that way.

Exercise Bubbles meditation – uncovering the Self

This is really a guided visualization rather than meditation and is designed to reveal the Self. The exercise is easier if it is read to you. However, a much better way is to read through the instructions, understand them, and then do it on your own, using your own will rather than someone else's.

Find a comfortable, seated position on the floor or in a chair. If you can maintain 'the force' throughout you will be doing well.

Become aware of your physical sensations. Take some time, do not get distracted by them, just be aware of exactly where your body is and of the sensations coming from your feet... lower legs... knees... thighs... hips... spine... neck... shoulders... arms... hands... head... face... neck... front of you body... any parts missed out. Become aware of all these sensations and put a bubble around them. Place the bubble away from you so that your consciousness is outside of it.

Now become aware of your feelings – the feelings you have at this moment, about doing what you are doing. Do not let them suck you in, just maintain an objective view of all your feelings. Put a bubble around them and place them away from your consciousness. Give yourself (or the person to whom you are reading this) the necessary time to complete this part.

Now become aware of your thoughts – the thoughts you are having at this moment, thoughts you have had in the last few minutes. Do not get stuck on them, just view them objectively. Put a bubble around them and place them away from consciousness. Allow sufficient time for this.

You have separated yourself from your body, feelings and thoughts and now have the opportunity to be aware of your Self. You may be able to notice how it is beyond time, is infinite in size, yet contains something you may call love or peace. Stay here for a while.

To finish, you need to reverse the process. First, bring back into your consciousness, the bubble that contains your thoughts... next, bring back feelings... and now bring back physical sensations. (If you are reading this to someone or directing them, notice how they change as each bubble is brought back.) Finally, slowly open your eyes.

Reversing the process makes it easier to practise the meditation next time.

Moving to 'heaven' from the Self, as with the movement to Self from 'earth', can only be achieved through working with the life force. This can be made possible through meditation, yoga, prayer, the arts, religion and a million other ways but not through science. Science is incredibly limited since it only uses 'thoughts'. Science, leaves feelings aside, but to be able to move from 'earth' to 'heaven' you need to know feelings.

Exercise Meditation resolution

> *Resolve to meditate daily. Write this intention in your journal. If you do not currently meditate daily, I would recommend that you start with only two minutes each day. I know this doesn't sound like a lot but you need to establish the pattern first without experiencing the difficulties. In the second week, extend it to three minutes. What you want to avoid is doing five minutes or more one day and then saying to yourself on the following day, 'I did enough yesterday; I don't need to do it today.' Always make changes in small amounts and remember that the idea of meditation is to bring into focus the elements of your self which you normally do not want to look at. If your meditation starts to get difficult, you know that it is working.*

Meditation is a natural act that we have somehow forgotten to accommodate in our busy lives. It probably happened more readily when there was no electricity. Being aware of the pitfalls that you may encounter along the way is important. For example, your ego will go to amazing lengths to stop you meditating: marvellous events, essential tasks and interesting television programmes will present themselves just as you were about to sit. One way around this problem is to have a regular time each day when you meditate and then to stick to it absolutely, regardless of what else happens. However, this requires effort which, as I said before, in the long term is unsustainable unless you use it to overcome inertia – that is precisely what you are doing here.

Summary

Eight steps to health, happiness and enlightenment

Record your steps in a journal.

Find and maintain 'the force' throughout your daily activities.

Exercise: *both stretching and aerobic, maintaining awareness of 'the force' and using no more effort than is required to overcome initial inertia.*

Diet: *develop food sensitivity awareness and follow the guidance of your own life force.*

Yoga *(the science of resolving inner conflict): Salute to the Sun, Maha Mudra.*

Pranayama: *developing energy flow with breathing exercises.*

Mudras: *focusing awareness in different areas.*

Mantras and affirmations: *to clear out inner conflict.*

Miracles and magic: *realizing your power and letting go of those things which you think you own.*

Meditation: *also to clear inner conflict. Start with less; leave yourself wanting more.*

Part 5: The Boulderstone Technique of Life Force Healing

The quickest way to enlightenment and perfect health

There is a fast route to enlightenment but, as with all fast routes, there are dangers attached. For that reason, I highly recommend that if you want to pursue this route you find someone who knows how to deal with the associated problems that come with it.

You will be enlightened when you can stay with 'the force' regardless of what difficulties there are. Learning how to do this is your objective. Problems arise because it is difficult to get an objective view of what is going on for us; however, there is a way round this. The solution is to help other people move to that state.

When a person uses the Boulderstone Technique to heal another person, they become one energetically. This allows the healer to see the other person's problems without the emotional baggage of the patient. The healer gets firsthand knowledge of how people heal. This is a fantastic learning opportunity for the healer.

In fact, there are only a limited number of problems in the world; helping other people overcome their problems is a perfect way to learn about them and how to overcome them. Healing other people teaches you how the life force works and could be the biggest single aid to your spiritual development. Of course, not everyone wants to help others but, if you do, you will learn rapidly.

Exercise *Tune into another person and get 'the force'. It is best if they are lying down on their back with your hands cradling their head. Check how you are currently feeling. Ask them to think about a current problem they have and see how your feelings change. Do not try and do anything; just bear witness to what is happening to you and the patient.*

Change roles, so that 'patient' becomes 'practitioner'.

The Boulderstone Technique

Up until now, all therapies have had a structure. This has been required for diagnosis to occur. Western medicine has the body systems, acupuncture has the meridians, Ayurvedic medicine has the chakras. However, the Boulderstone Technique of Life Force Healing is different; it does not define a human being. It says that if you are ill then you are the one who has created a limiting structure; this limiting structure is the sole cause of your illness. This includes every condition that causes you pain in any way.

The Boulderstone Technique works with the energetic structure which has been created, finds its inner conflict and addresses it. A practitioner does not impose any of their own ideas on the person; there are no moral judgements. However, advice on lifestyle and food choices is often given, especially if the patient is unaware of their own life force. As a Boulderstone Technique practitioner, you work with what is presented, not with what you think is there. Symptom descriptions actually become unimportant as far as the healing is concerned, because you actually feel what is happening in the vitality of the patient, through your hands, and thus get to the cause of the problem. This cause is always inner conflict. When the inner conflict is resolved, the patient is better.

Removing a block

Knowing how to remove an energetic block is probably the single most important thing you need to learn in this life. Everyone has done it. Even if you appear to get cured through taking pills, somewhere along the way you must have employed your *I-force* and life force to remove the block.

While it is true that everyone knows how to remove blocks, not everyone knows how to remove them consciously.

When a block is removed you end up with emptiness. You can experience what this means by staring at a candle. After a while, even though your eyes are open and you are looking at it, in a sense you cannot see it anymore. It hasn't disappeared but you are looking at its essential nature – emptiness. The same thing happens when you are in a quiet room with a ticking clock. After a while, you become so used to the ticking that you cannot hear it any more. The clock hasn't stopped ticking but you have gone beyond the noise to its essential nature. Of course, you can tune back into the ticking at any time, if you want to.

Now, it just so happens that, if you isolate anything and stay focused on it whilst at the same time remaining aware of what you are doing, then that thing, whatever it is, will disappear for you. In order to stay focused you need to use your *I-force:* to stay aware you need to be able to follow your life force.

This holds true for things as disparate as, say, a tune that has got stuck in your head or the grief you feel for a dead relative. It allows you to see the essential nature of the 'object' you are looking at. But you must focus on what I call the energy of the 'object'. In the case of the tune, this is just the tune in your head; in the case of the bereavement it is the 'pain' of the grief. The reason a tune stays stuck in your head is that you do not allow it to complete; you either lose awareness or try to cut it off – you use either too little *I-force* or too much. These are the only reasons why a tune will get stuck. The same is true for grief or any other mental/emotional problem, including panic attacks and other anxieties.

So, the method for removing any block is to use energetically-focused awareness. All successful therapies boil down to this. If you remove all your blocks, you will be left in complete health. You do not need to do anything else. Because this is cure, when it is completed, not only do the symptoms disappear but the patient often forgets that they ever had them. Can you remember all the illnesses you have ever had? Of course not, they have been cured on a fundamental level. Unfortunately, this memory loss is what makes it possible to dismiss the cure as trivial. For example, the patient may say, 'I was getting better anyway,' or, 'Time is a great healer.' It is not time that is the great healer, but the life force which is working all the time. Patients forget how much the healer has helped, too.

Being able to focus on the energy of a problem and stay aware is the way to remove all blocks. Words are not needed, homeopathic remedies are not needed, acupuncture needles are not needed, herbs are not needed – although all of these things can help to focus awareness. What is needed is an understanding of the structure the patient has built up which, in turn, causes symptoms. Structures are built by the patient with *I-force*. The healer recreates the structure and the patient dismantles it, thus allowing the life force to flow freely. In this way, all blocks can be removed and with them all illnesses. Every illness, whether diagnosed or not, can be treated – there are no exceptions.

Symptoms are truly the signposts to enlightenment.

Acknowledgements

How many people does it take to write a book? In my case not many but without any of these people mentioned here this book would not have happened. At the end of the day a book is just a collection of paper with a few scribbles on them; however, during the process of writing there were times when these sheets of paper became the most important thing in my world while at other times it was a source of pain and grief. Perhaps it is the same with all things you believe you create.

Chantal Roser made more suggestions than I thought there were ideas in the book, her assistance was invaluable. Katharine, my wife, helped with words, ideas and suggestions and by giving me the space to write and think. Amber and Zoë, my daughters, through being themselves and willing to explore aspects of the life force.

Many thanks to Tim Roser and Christian for their help with the illustrations.

Paul Smith helped in my development and understanding of what I call the I-force.

Without the positive feedback from my patients and students I would never have developed what has become known as the Boulderstone Technique.

The greatest thanks, however, has to go to the Life Force. As this force is culturally independent but our starting points are not, gratitude is due to the Holy Spirit, Lord Shiva, Kundalini, Ruach, the Tao, Chi, Prana et al.

Contact details

For courses in the Boulderstone Technique of Life Force Healing, treatment or more information you can contact us either via e-mail living@life-force-healing.co.uk or by phone 08456-443626 or look at the website www.boulderstonetechnique.com

If you like the ideas presented here please help spread them by buying another copy of this book and giving it to a friend or colleague. Your life force is the unifying link which will allow every health-poor person to become rich again.

With love, John

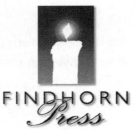

FINDHORN
Press

To obtain a copy of the current Findhorn Press catalogue please contact us by email: info@findhornpress.com
or phone: 01309 690582.

Alternatively, please visit our website: www.findhornpress.com